FUN
FITNESS TRAINING
FOR KIDS

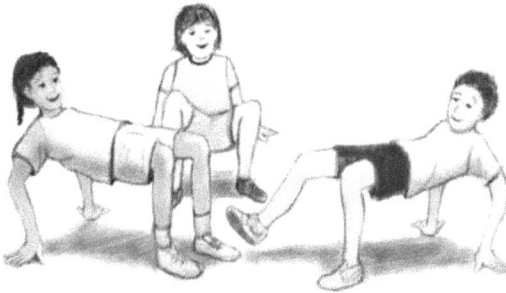

Everything you need to know
to get your kids in shape while having fun!

Sue Tracey

In Collaboration with Jane Eyre

"For all those who don't feel as old as they are,
and never will."

Jimmy Buffett

Michael:

You're the best thing that ever happened to me!

Sue

Text © 2010 Sue Tracey

Book Design & Illustrations © 2010 Jane Eyre

ISBN 978 - 0 - 615 - 35686 - 0

DISCLAIMER

The content, techniques and suggestions in this book are not intended as a substitute for consultations with a medical professional. All forms of exercise can pose some inherent risks. Please be advised to take full responsibility for protecting first and foremost the physical well-being of children. Never take risks beyond a child's experience, training, and fitness

TABLE OF CONTENTS

INTRODUCTION

This book contains fun activities and games that will challenge children to improve their muscular strength, muscular endurance, flexibility, coordination, speed, agility, power, balance, and aerobic endurance for overall fitness. It can be used as a handbook by parents, youth group leaders, coaches, teachers, and more.

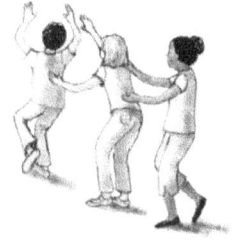

THE IMPORTANCE OF PHYSICAL ACTIVITY FOR CHILDREN

The US Health & Human Services recommends children have at least 60 minutes of physical activity a day. The 60 minutes does not have to be continuous.

Children who do exercise are more likely to lower their risks of many health problems, increase bone mineral density, sleep better, have less anxiety, gain self-efficacy, and a better self image.

Exercise helps most of the body's systems perform at an optimal level.

It also is important to know that children who are unfit have a very high percentage rate of becoming obese or adults who are not physically fit.

The **KEEP IT SIMPLE (KIS)** principle is used throughout this book.

Take some time and read through pages 6 through 17 to study how to correctly perform the exercises and stretches ... then go out and have fun with the activities!

BEFORE YOU START

BE AWARE OF SAFETY

Whenever you have movement, you increase the chance of injury. Always be aware of potential dangers inside or outside before starting any activity, such as slippery surfaces, uneven surfaces, furniture, toys, fences, clothing, family pets, trees, etc.

- If the hazards can be removed, do so; when not, they need to be marked off with cones or lines.

- Visually show and verbally warn children of the high-risk or off-limit areas.

- When playing, they should have proper clothing, shoes, and gear.

- Before beginning any vigorous activities, warming-up the muscles and joints helps prevent injuries.

THE LEARNING PROCESS

A child does not have to be an athlete to enjoy exercise and activity. When a child participates in any athletic endeavor, they will improve with practice. Some children think failure is final; it is not! Children often will stay motivated and strive to do their best if they compete against themselves rather than against others. Encouraging their little accomplishments often will help a child spur on their efforts to do better.

- Be sensitive to children's weaknesses or special needs by adapting rules to fit their needs.

- If you want them to do their best, do not embarrass or harass them.

- Have fun and present the activity enthusiastically.

- Your body language, enthusiasm, voice, and, sense of humor all help lead a child to having fun with fitness.

- Children have different ways of comprehending rules. Try to present games using visual, auditory, and kinesthetic methods.

- Preschoolers have limited attention spans and cannot grasp complex games. Spatial awareness also is difficult to understand.

- Some children from ages 6 to 9 understand complex games, but others cannot stay focused and have no idea what is going on.

- Children from ages 10 to 12 can play games that have many rules and various skills.

- Try to encourage the child to face difficult tasks as challenges .

ASSESSING THE FITNESS OF A CHILD

Exercise will increase a child's fitness level. By making fitness assessments you can help identify the rate of progress. All of the activities in this book can be performed at a moderate intensity that is not dangerous. If a child is obese or has other physical limitations a physician should be consulted.

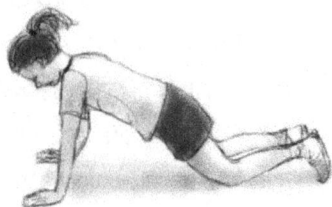

The body needs appropriate amounts of fat and lean tissue for optimal health. The Body Mass Index (BMI) is a fairly simple means of measuring the proportion of fat versus lean tissue. The Centers for Disease Control and Prevention (CDC) has a BMI Percentile Calculator for Children on their website www.cdc.gov. You need to know the child's birth date, date of measurement, sex, height to nearest 1/8 inch, and their weight to nearest ¼ pound. Do not use an adult BMI calculator to measure a child.

The President's Challenge www.presidentschallenge.org has a Physical Fitness Test that often is given in schools. The test consists of curl-ups, shuttle-run, endurance run/walk, pull-ups or right angle pushups, and the v-sit or sit and reach.

Each child is unique and wellness check-ups vary for different children and issues. Children should have a good physical exam by a pediatrician before getting involved in physical training.

INJURIES

WHEN IN DOUBT CALL 911!

In many cases the **RICE** method (Rest, Ice, Compression and Elevation) should be used immediately after an injury occurs.

- ***REST**-do not use the injured part

- ***ICE-** apply ice to the area for 20 minutes. Keep re-applying ice every 2 to 6 hours for 2 days

- ***COMPRESSION-** to prevent further swelling, wrap the injury, but do not cut off circulation

- ***ELEVATION**-place injured area higher than the heart to help drain fluids away from injury.

HEAD AND SPINAL CORD INJURIES should be handled by medical experts; **CALL 911 IMMEDIATELY** and do not move victim.

HEAT RELATED ILLNESSES: Active exercising in hot conditions can cause heat cramps, heat exhaustion and heat stroke. Heat exhaustion and heat cramps can usually be relieved with rest, plenty of water and a cool environment.

If you think the child is having a heat stroke (very high body temperature, flush skin and not currently sweating) call 911 immediately. Check the airways for breathing, move the child to a cooler environment, remove clothing, and try to cool the body down by placing ice packs in the armpits, groin, and neck while waiting for help.

TRAINING

TRAINING TIPS

- Master the move before going on to the next level. Example: Start with modified plank. If the child can hold this move for 30 seconds, rest, and then try the upward plank for 10 to 30 seconds.

- Modify rest between activities depending on need.

- Progress with stable moves before attempting unstable moves.
  Example:
  1. Two leg squat
  2. Two leg squat with upper body movement
  3. One leg squat
  4. One leg squat with upper body movement

- Be aware of environmental conditions: heat, cold, humidity, wetness, and wind.

- Monitor all participants.

- Whenever possible try to have child face away from the sun. Objects are difficult to see with the sun shining into their eyes.

- Set a good example and include fitness in your life.

- Warm-up the body before exercising and cool-down at the end of the session.

- Put less stress on joints. When moving feet have "soft" i.e., not tense, knees and hips on landing.

- To improve balance and symmetry, be sure to work both sides equally when performing an exercise that requires a single leg or arm or starting with a specific side. Be sure to switch sides.

- Children should not hold their breath during a workout, breathing helps one exercise productively.

- Think variety: up - down, left - right, forward - backward, diagonal, slow - fast, big - small, balanced and off balanced movements.

- The average child grows 2 or more inches a year and does not always know where their body starts or ends.

- Before doing a plyometric exercise, make sure balance, stability, and proper form are established.

- Do not work through pain; if an exercise hurts... stop doing it.

- To change directions when moving from one space to another a child needs to decelerate before accelerating.

- When in a safe area, warming up in bare feet can help strengthen the ankle support system.

- If child cannot go all the way down while performing a push-up or modified push-up, have them go half way down and all the way up or half way up and then down.

- Encourage the child to "smile" when exercising.

- SOM: Progress slow to fast.

- ROM: Start with small movements and progress to large movements.

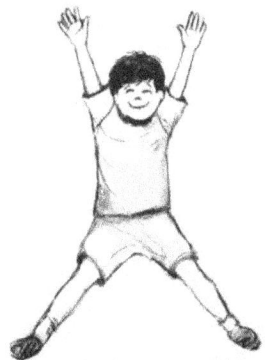

- With fatigue, skill and balance can diminish.

- If in doubt of fitness or skill level, start with a single/simple challenge and gradually work to complex / multitask challenges.
  For example:
    - Hop on one foot up and down
    - Hop on one foot side to side
    - Hop on one foot side to side and hold a Weighted tennis ball
    - Hop on one foot side to side swinging a weighted tennis ball up and down

- Never participate outside when you hear thunder.

- Never assume the child understands exactly what to do.

- Stay positive by saying "you are doing great" or "keep going" instead of "don't quit".

- Make sure the child is eating nutritious food and staying hydrated throughout the day.

- Don't dwell on mistakes, learn from them.

- Keep in mind the "FITT" Principle. FREQUENCY, INTENSITY, TIME & TYPE of exercise.

- Add a twist (rotation) and/or balance activity to work the core.

- **Have fun, have fun, have fun!**

QUANTIFYING INTENSITY

How hard someone feels they are working can be a reliable guide to aerobic intensity.

One test is the **"TALK TEST."** The inability to talk is a sign of too much intensity.

Another test is the "**BORG SCALE"**. Participants are asked what number they perceive or the way they feel while exercising. Rating of Perceived Exertion (RPE) is a subjective means of estimating exercise intensity.

The BORG 6 to 20 RPE Scale:

6 No exertion at all

7 Extremely light

8

9 Very light

10

11 Light

12

13 Somewhat hard

14

15 Hard (heavy)

16

17 Very hard

18

19 Extremely hard

20 Maximal exertion

Borg. G. (1998). Borg's Perceived Exertion and Pain Scales. Champaign: IL: Human Kinetics

THE BODY AND MOVEMENT

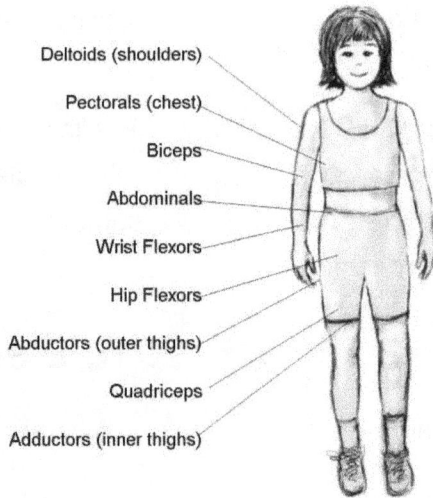

Deltoids (shoulders)
Pectorals (chest)
Biceps
Abdominals
Wrist Flexors
Hip Flexors
Abductors (outer thighs)
Quadriceps
Adductors (inner thighs)

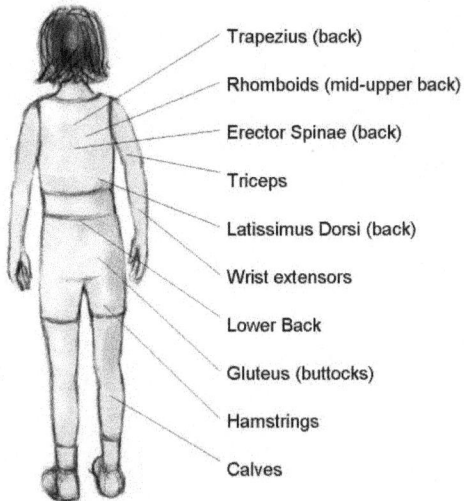

Trapezius (back)
Rhomboids (mid-upper back)
Erector Spinae (back)
Triceps
Latissimus Dorsi (back)
Wrist extensors
Lower Back
Gluteus (buttocks)
Hamstrings
Calves

MUSCLES, FASCIA, BONES, AND NERVES

Movement involves the skeletal, nervous, and muscular systems.

The muscular system is affected the most from exercise. There are over 600 muscles in the human body and a band of fibrous connective tissue that supports, covers, and separates all the muscle groups called fascia. Joint movement requires the fascia and several muscles take action in various ways. In fact, hundreds of muscles may play roles when performing one movement and this movement can affect the fascia at another end of the body (example: moving the right arm could affect the fascia in the left foot). When a muscle works, it may lengthen (eccentric contraction), stay the same (isometric contraction), or shorten in length (concentric contraction). The heart is also a muscle and exercise is very beneficial for it.

Muscle fatigue can be caused by various reasons: power moves, heavy exercise, or prolonged endurance activities.

Exercise enhances feedback from the nervous system. Reaction time, coordination, balance, and muscle memory, can all be improved through repeated exercise.

The skeleton consists of 206 bones in an adult. Children start with more than 206 bones, and the bones fuse as the child grows. The skeleton's main function in movement is to act as levers and support the body. The bones also protect organs and produce blood cells.

NEUTRAL SPINE

Many exercises should be done with a neutral spine/correct posture. To check posture, stand with heels, buttocks, shoulders, and head against a wall. Feel the space in the arch of the back with a hand. There should be just enough room for one hand to slide between the arch and the wall. Many people need to be reminded about their posture when exercising, standing, or sitting.

BALANCE

Performing activities that require balance helps activate many reflex actions. Anything from a small shift of weight in the toes to moving the shoulders, involves the stabilizing muscles trying to hold the center of gravity.

CORE STRENGTH

Core strength refers to the muscles of the lower back, abdominals, hips, and pelvis and their ability to support and balance the body. In healthy individuals, activation of the core muscles occurs before any movement of the body or a body segment.

Activating or engaging the core is done by contracting the pelvic muscles as if trying to stop from urinating and by pulling in the lower belly.

Unstable exercises and trying to regain or maintain posture usually work the core more than a crunch exercise.

EXERCISES

WARMING UP

Always warm-up. Warming-up muscles will make them pliable and is known to improve co-ordination and reaction time. It prepares the muscles and the joints for more intense activity.

A warm-up can be as simple as marching in place and moving the arms in circles or doing a slow, less intense version of the activity that you are about to perform.

You want the warm-up slowly to increase the heart rate.

AEROBIC EXERCISES

Aerobic exercise is any exercise that increases the body's demand for oxygen over an extended time. Aerobic activity puts demands on the cardiovascular and respiratory systems to function at a higher level of performance. Jogging laps is boring for most children. Aerobic exercise is more enjoyable when you mix-up the aerobic movements or play a game that involves a variety of movements over a period of time. Aerobic movement can be performed in one location (i.e: marching in place).

Aerobic Movement Examples: jogging, running, hopping, marching, walking at various speeds, jumping, jump roping, swimming, bicycling, stair climbing, skipping, side shuffle, dancing, jogging heels high in the back, jogging knees high in the front, jumping jacks, leaping, back pedaling, and MORE.

BASIC EXERCISE POSITIONS

In this book, some exercises will be repeated in different ways because they are some of the best body strengthening exercises a child can do. In some cases there are easier versions of the exercise. As a child becomes stronger, encourage the more difficult version.

Look at the charts to see each progression. The harder version versus the easier version (modified) is a good way of equalizing different abilities when performing activities against someone stronger or weaker.

To help prevent injury and to get the most out of an exercise, proper body alignment is important. Before a child does an exercise, study the diagrams and instructions.

SQUAT: Increasing strength in the legs and buttocks.

Stand with feet just outside shoulder width, slightly angled outwards. Knees and hips are "soft" or slightly flexed. Activate the core and slowly push the hips back, bend the knees and lean forward with a straight back. Slowly raise the arms for balance. Hold and slowly press the body back up to the starting position.

- To modify all of the squats, do a shallow knee bend.

- One legged squats can be performed with the support of a prop or without support.

- **Important:** For all squats, do not have the knees extend beyond the toes or lower hips below knees during the bending motion.

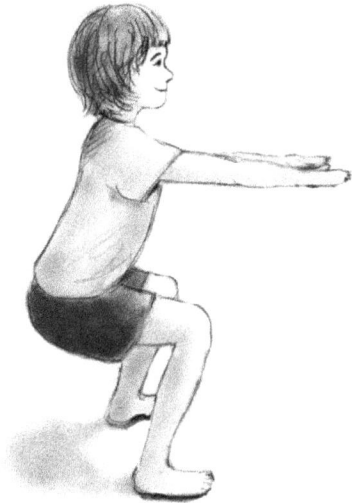

Squat

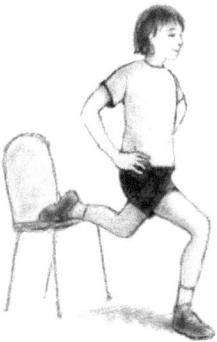

One - leg Posterior Squat

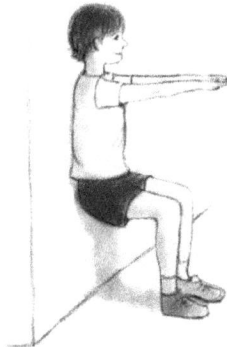

Wall Squat

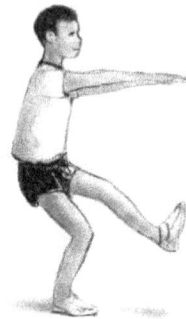

One - leg Anterior Squat
(This is difficult)

19

V-SEAT: A core balance exercise that builds abdominal muscles along with the supporting muscles of the lower back.

To increase intensity:
- Move arms and / or legs
- Lean to the right side with arms extended above the head
- Lean to the left side with both arms extended to the right

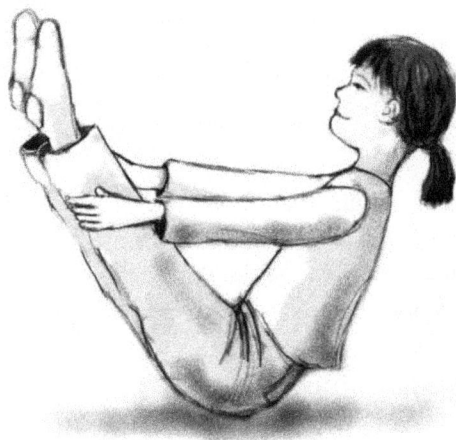

Sit on ground with knees slightly bent and legs slightly apart. Engage the core and lift the legs off the ground and place hands next to the knees or up in the air. Lean back slightly, straighten legs and balance the body on the tailbone so that legs and torso will form the letter "V". Try to hold this position. If unable to do this, modify by lowering the leg lift and bending legs.

PUSH-UP: Involves the chest, shoulders, upper back and arm muscles. To increase intensity, put hands closer together under the chest or raise one limb off the ground.

Full Push-Up

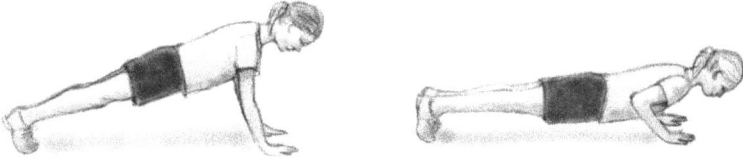

Lie with feet together, legs straight, toes tucked under feet in a prone position. The hands are flat on the ground under the shoulders. Straighten the arms and push the body off the floor. Keep the body straight and exhale while going up. Pause at the upward push-up position and then slowly bend arms and bring chest down to the ground. Inhale as the body goes down and do not allow knees to touch the ground or body to arch.

Raised Push-Up

Feet are on the ground and hands are on sturdy raised area. The body is straight and a full push-up is performed.

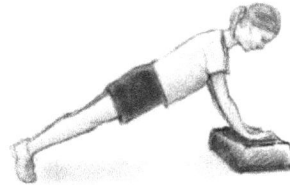

Modified Push-Up

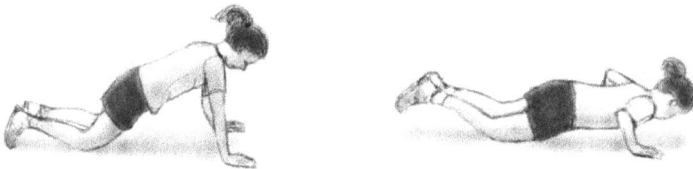

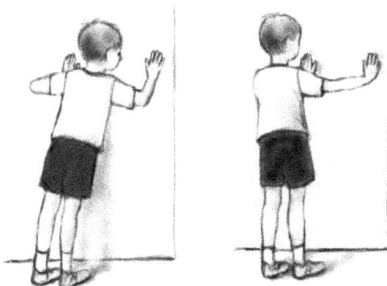

Wall Push-Up
(Easiest)   21

PLANK: Exercise for the whole body. The core muscles are used along with the arms and upper body.

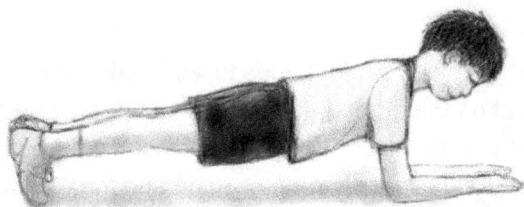

Lay on floor in a prone position. The only parts of the body that will be touching the ground will be the toes, forearms, and hands. Looking down, engage the core and lift the body up with forearms on the floor, elbows aligned under shoulders, fingers pointing away from body, palms flat on the ground, and toes on floor. Hold this position.

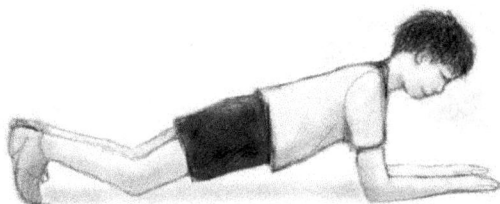

Modified Plank

LUNGE: Strengthens leg muscles, hips and buttocks. Also uses some of the upper body to help stabilize. Small and large steps in the lunge work the muscles in different ways. Small steps isolate the quadriceps and large steps work the hamstrings and buttocks.

For all lunges: Do not extend knees beyond toes

To perform an **ANTERIOR LUNGE**, stand with feet shoulder width apart, in a neutral spine position. Keeping the head up, step forward with the right leg, lowering until the right thigh is parallel with the floor. The back leg dips towards the floor.

The **POSTERIOR LUNGE** can be performed by moving the left leg back and ending in the same position as the anterior lunge.

For a **LATERAL LUNGE**, toes face forward, step to the right side and squat down by lowering the hips. The left leg will be straight to the side and the right knee will be bent forward. Keep both feet flat on the ground.

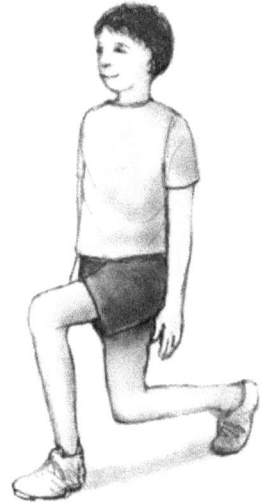

Anterior Lunge

FENCER'S LUNGE

Stand sideways, feet shoulder width apart, the front foot is facing forward and back foot facing outwards at a 90 degree angle and arms down at sides. Kick the front leg forward and at the same time reach the front arm forward, back arm pushes backwards and back leg straightens. The front foot lands on the heel first and then the rest of the foot rocks forward to land. The front knee is bent directly over the heel, back leg is straight with the foot flat on the ground, and the weight is evenly distributed over both feet.

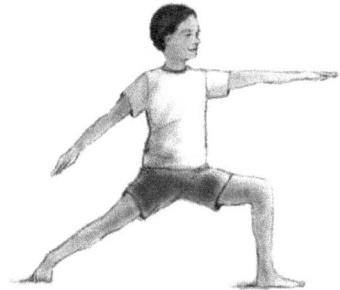

23

BIRD - DOG: A great exercise for the core body.

Start on hands and knees with knees directly below hips, hands below shoulders and looking downward. Activate core and slowly raise straight arm and opposite straight leg without losing posture or balance. Hold for 10 seconds or more.

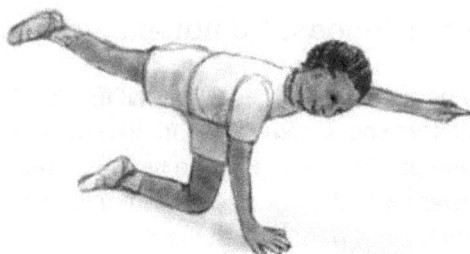

To modify this exercise, just hold one arm out and then a leg.

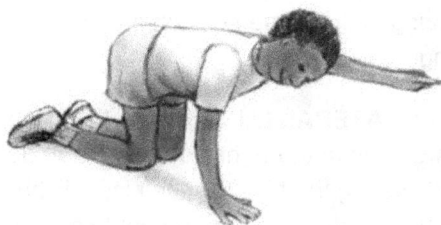

One arm out

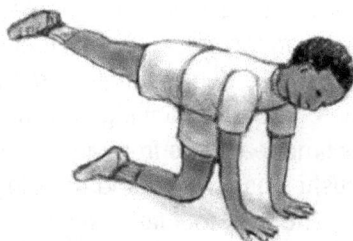

One leg up

CRAB: Targets shoulders, arms, legs, and the core

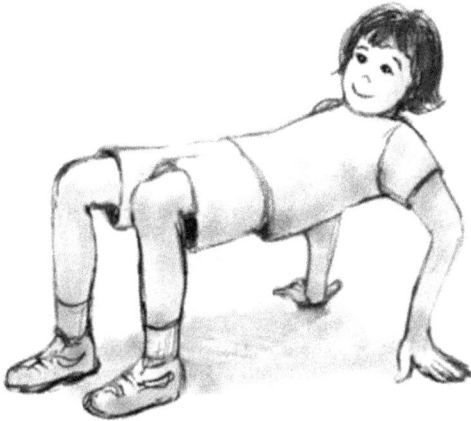

Sit on ground with knees bent, feet flat, and place palms on the ground near upper hips. Make the body look like a table by lifting up the hips making the torso the tabletop with the arms and legs being the legs of the table. Hands should be directly under the shoulders and feet under the knees. The crab exercise can be performed by staying stationary, walking forward, backward, or sideways and doing slight dips by bending arms. To intensify, lift opposite foot and hand at the same time and hold.

STRETCHING

Flexibility and balance are an important part of fitness. Many of the yoga poses help improve range of motion, flexibility, balance, strength and muscular efficiency. The body should be warmed-up before attempting a stretch.

With yoga poses, try to relax the body as much as possible, breath, and do not bounce. Hold the static poses 5 to 30 seconds, rest and repeat movement."

Most children have an interest in doing yoga. If you have a child who is not quite sure and might think it is a feminine exercise, let them know that many professional athletes participate in yoga.

The following are some yoga moves that children enjoy. Before the children perform the move tell them the name of the pose. The imagery of the name helps children enjoy it more.

HAPPY BABY: This is a V-Seat with legs wide apart and your right hand grabbing your right foot and left hand grabbing left foot ... rock gently, side to side or forward and backward. SMILE !

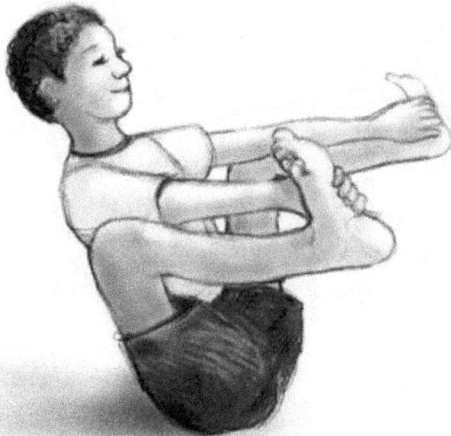

TRIANGLE: Stand with feet wide apart with your right foot pointed forward and left foot turned at about 90 degrees to the side. Bend down the left side and reach the left hand down left leg as close to ankle as possible. Stretch right arm up towards the ceiling and look at the right hand. Release the position slowly and repeat on the other side.

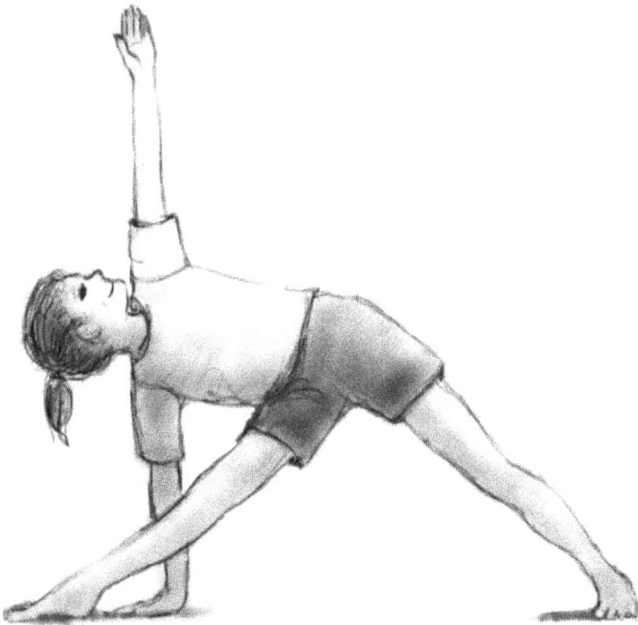

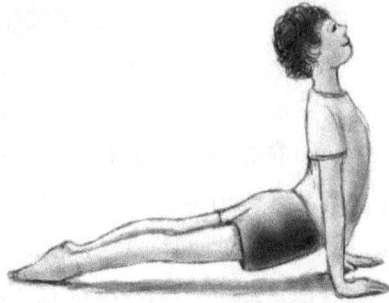

UPWARD DOG: In the downward pushup position with the top of feet against the floor. Slowly straighten arms and look up toward the sky. Lift so the hips and legs are slightly off the floor. The tops of feet and hands will be the only thing touching the floor. Using arms, slowly come back down to the original position.

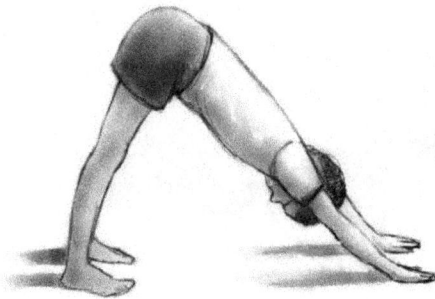

DOWNWARD DOG: Get down on hands and knees. Keeping the palms of hands and the balls of feet touching the floor, slowly straighten legs and bring butt up high into the air and tuck chin down. This forms an upside down V. Now, slowly bring heels as close to the ground as possible. Hold this position and then slowly release out of it.

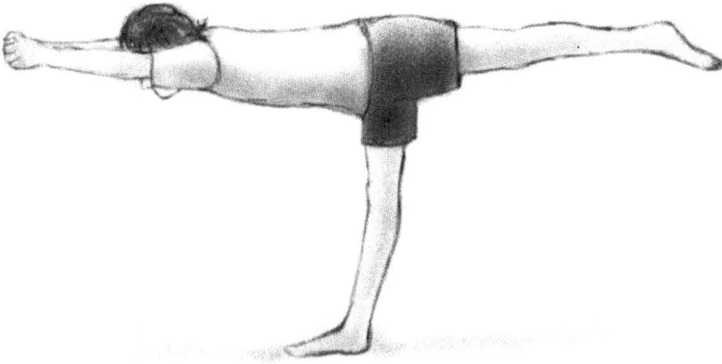

BALANCE STICK POSE: Stand with feet together, arms are straight up over the head, biceps pressed against ears, palms together, and fingers straight. Take a big step forward with right leg and point left toe behind. In one straight movement from fingers to left toes, raise left leg behind and arms down in front, keeping the head between arms and the right leg straight. From the side, the body will look like the letter "T". This is a very challenging pose. Encourage the efforts to keep trying and to add seconds to the hold each time

WARRIOR I & WARRIOR II: Think strong and proud for both of the Warrior positions. Do a right and then left lunge.

Warrior I is a lunge position with front foot facing forward and back foot at a 90 degree angle. Arms go straight up in the air with palms facing inward.
Look upward or straight ahead.

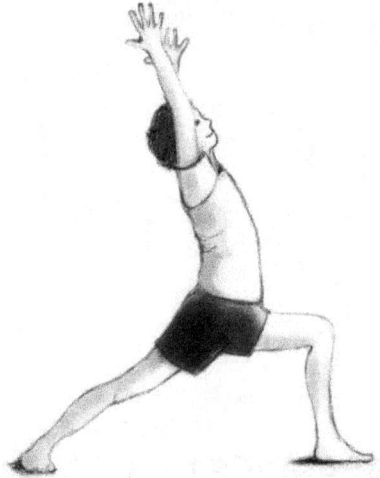

Warrior II is also done in the same lunge position except the arms are extended out to your sides with palms down. Look toward the extended arm over the bent leg.

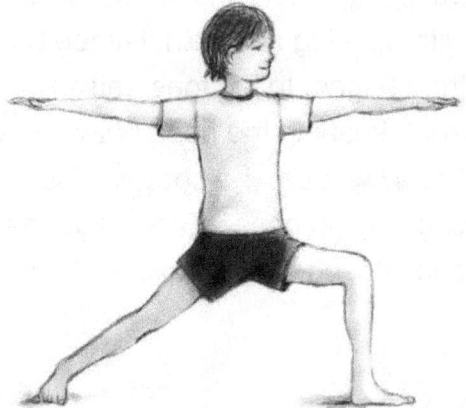

MOUNTAIN POSE: Standing very tall with feet together and arms hanging at side with palms facing the body. Feel like someone is pulling the top of head towards the ceiling and the whole body is lengthening.

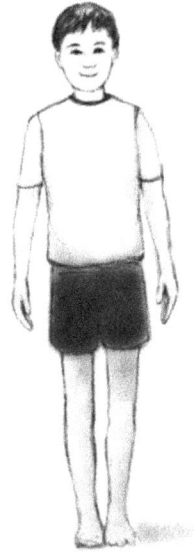

CRESCENT MOON: Standing in the mountain pose, reach left arm up toward the sky, palm facing inward and spread fingers. Keep reaching upwards and slowly bend over to the right, hold, come back up to center, and then bend to the left.

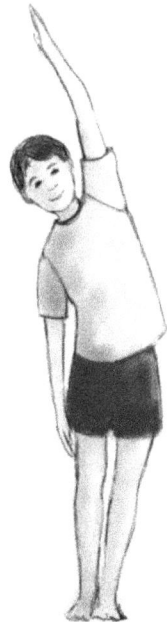

OSTRICH POSE: With feet wide apart, reach arms up and then fold down forward slowly. Try to place hands on the floor or place on legs and look between legs. Slowly come back up.

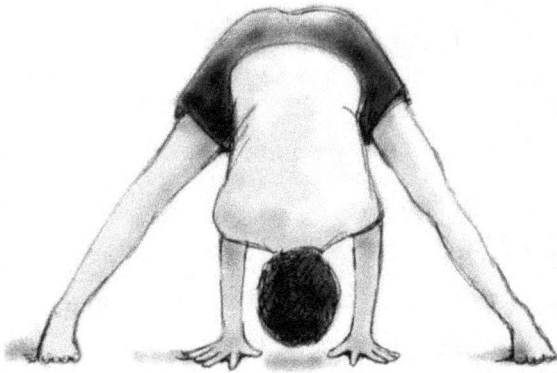

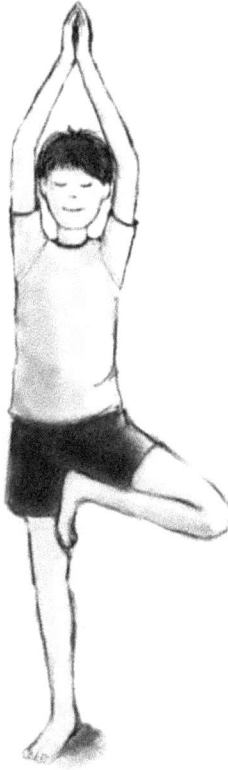

TREE POSE: Think of one foot grounded into the earth and standing firm. Begin by standing in the mountain pose and put palms together in front of chest prayer style. Bring left foot up and try to place left sole on inner right thigh. Modify this by placing the sole on the right calf, even easier is placing the sole on the right foot. When balanced, slowly bring the arms up over the head with the palms still together. HOLD....and then start over with other leg.

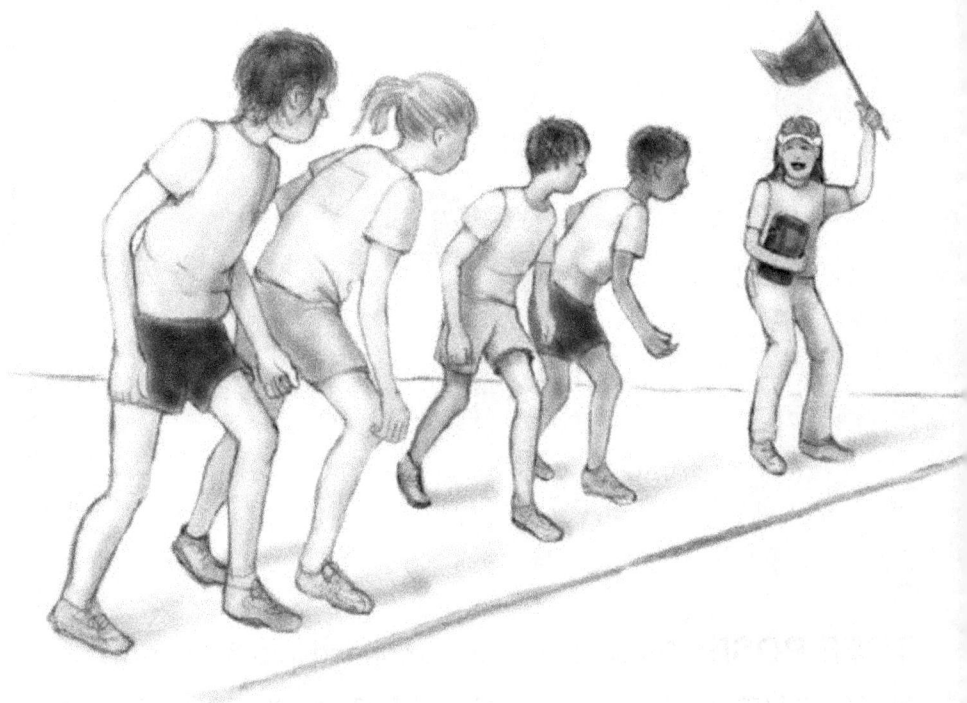

LET'S GET STARTED!

When doing activities with several children it helps to have a signal (whistle/hand clap) to immediately stop. Let them know that when the whistle blows or the lights blink they are to stop moving. One way to practice this is to have children move slowly around the play area and when the stop motion signal is given, they freeze like a statue. Praising the child who was quick to freeze also is an incentive for others to do the same.

- Many of the activities can be done in a large or small area. When in a small area, change fast movements to marching, walking with knees high, lunge walking, choo-choo steps (tiny fast shuffling), or crab walking.

- Have children make mini medicine balls or hand weights out of old tennis balls. Make a small slit and fill with little rocks, use a strong glue over slit and then tape on top of the glue. Keep away from the dog!

- Old socks are great to use as balls, boundary markers, in place of cones, or to use in tag games. The child also can also grab the ends of the sock with their hands and do stretching exercises.

FOR ONE OR MORE PARTICIPANTS

JACK IN THE BOX: Stand with feet shoulder width apart, very slowly squat down and when given a signal (hands clapped, whistle, lights flicker) jump up as high as possible and shout **"POP!!"**

POP!!

Option: For a more challenging plyometric move, have the child stand on the ground and jump onto a higher sturdy platform or step.

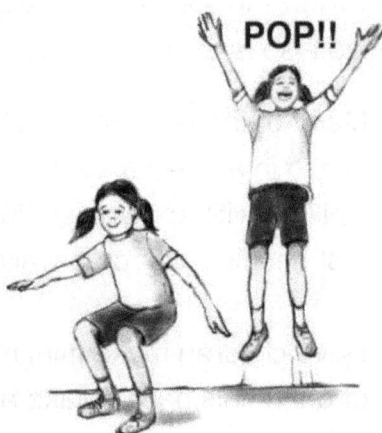

WALL WRITING: Stand arm's length away facing a wall with feet shoulder width apart. Hold a ball of socks or yarn ball with dominate hand, arm straight, and have the ball lightly touching the wall. Keep shoulders and hips square to wall. Use the ball to trace numbers starting with "1." How high up can they draw? Now try with other hand.

Option: To make this more challenging lift a foot off the ground or stand sideways to the wall and lift a foot off the ground.

BLASTOFF: Standing with right foot well in front, slowly go down into a lunge bending both legs. As they slowly descend count down 10, 9, 8, 7, 6, 5, 4, 3, 2, 1 then **"BLASTOFF".** With the word "blastoff", jump as high as possible and switch feet in the air so that the left foot is now in front when a soft landing is made. Now do the same with the left foot in front.

Option: A very challenging plyometric move is to have the child in the upright push-up position , slowly bend arms, and on "BLASTOFF", push-up quickly and try to push hands off the ground and have a soft landing ending in an upright push-up position.

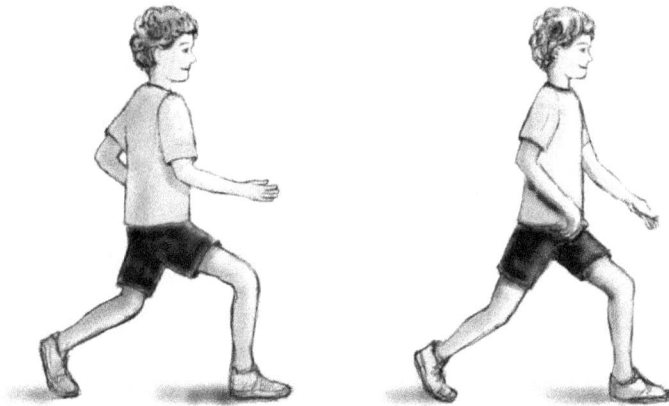

PUSH-UP PASS: In upright push-up position, have a sock, glove, yarn-ball, or beanbag under right hand. Push object to left while staying in the push-up position or downward dog position. Stop the object with the left hand and now push it back to the right.

Option:

- Perform in Ostrich Pose or Downward Dog
- After each pass perform a push-up

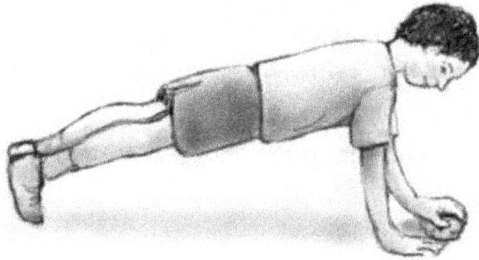

RACE CAR DRIVER: In an open space, set out several cones or markers in a zigzag pattern. Vary the space between markers 8 to 12 feet. Have little children pretend to start their engines and make "zoom" noises as they run and dodge the markers. Time the older children.

Option:

- Hold weighted tennis balls

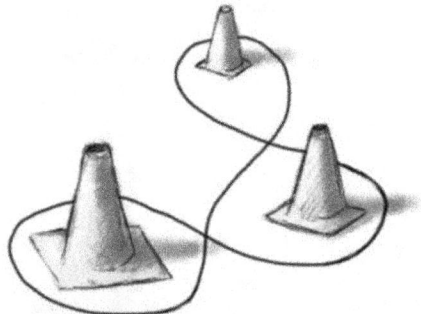

SIT TIGHT: Tell an action story and have seated children act out the movements while sitting.

Some suggestions:

- Walking down the street
- Riding a horse
- Jumping puddles
- Picking apples from a tree
- Chased by a skunk
- Skiing down a mountain
- Swimming across a pool
- Picking up heavy rocks
- Driving a tractor over a bumpy field
- Riding a bike
- Walking or running up and down a hill
- Climbing a ladder
- Surfing
- Climbing a tree and then hanging from a limb
- Walking on a tight rope

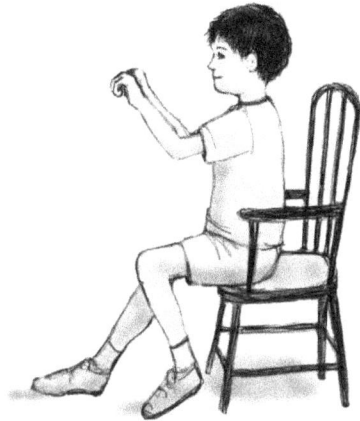

TV TIME: When watching TV, everyone can exercise.

- Marching in place while sitting on the sofa. Keep marching or walking during the whole show.

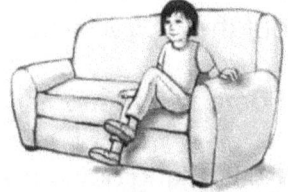

- Dance, march, jumping jacks, or jog during commercials.

- Stand up and sit down as many times as possible during a commercial.

- Pick a different exercise for every commercial.

- Lean back and quickly flutter-kick your legs like a swimmer when theme song is playing.

- Lay on floor and put legs up in the air. Pretend the ceiling is paper and the foot is a pen. Spell the names of favorite TV shows with right foot and then left foot.

- When show has ended put feet on chair or couch (no shoes) and put hands on floor. Stay in a raised foot plank or do pushups from this position.

- Put the channel changer across the room and crab walk to it when needed.

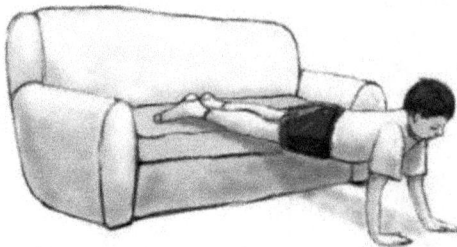

LIGHTS, CAMERA, ACTION: The child pretends to be an actor. Make cards with an action (marching, jumping, triangle pose, squats, etc.) and cards with an emotion (sad, excited, bored, etc.) and separate into two piles. The child selects a card from each pile and performs their action with emotion.

Examples:

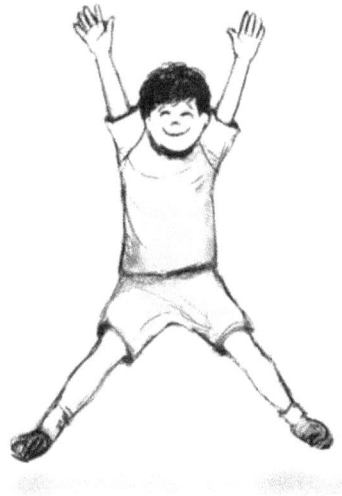

- Triangle Pose / Surprised

- Happy Baby Pose / Enthusiastic

- Ostrich Pose / Sad

- Jump / Joyfully

- Squat / Depressed

- Walk / Silly

- Run / Fearful

- Sit and Stand / Disappointed

- Tip-toe / Timidly

- March / Prideful

- Crabwalk / Happily

ANIMAL MOVEMENTS: This is for the young or young at heart. On command, the child will act out an animal. Have a signal for them to stop.

Some suggestions:
- Frog
- Crab (belly up, walking sideways)
- Alligator (low body and short legs)
- Kangaroo
- Monkey
- Bird
- Snake
- Inch worm (Upward push-up, walk feet to hands, and then walk feet back and hands forward
- Chicken

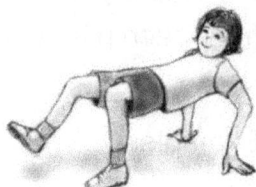

When you want the child to slow down try:
- Snail
- Frog on a lily pad
- Kitten sleeping
- Dead bug (on back with arms and legs straight up in the air
- Dog pointing (birddog)
- Bird in a nest
- Turtle.

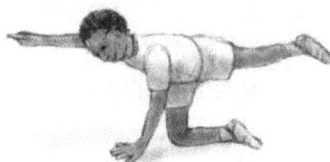

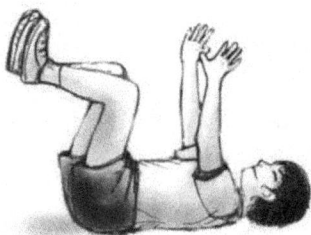

DANCE,DANCE,DANCE: Dancing is a great aerobic activity.

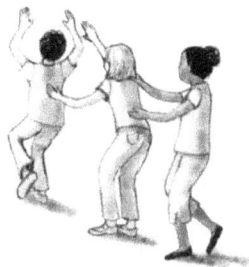

- Play a favorite song and make up a dance

- Make up a line dance

- Learn an old dance from a movie

- Sit and see how many dance moves can be done while sitting

- Think of a cartoon character and dance the way you think he/she/it would dance

- Dance in various exercise positions: squat, crab, pushup, V-seat

- Dribble a ball to music

- Hold socks or scarves in hands and shake up and down and all around

- While dancing keep one foot still on the ground, or both feet still

- Dance with one foot off the ground

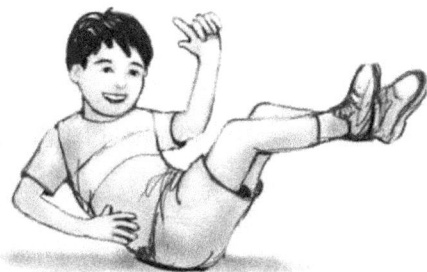

PILLOW POWER: Find two fairly firm pillows. The firmer the pillow the more difficult the balance exercise. Be careful not to twist ankles when balancing.

- Stand on one pillow with both feet and try not to fall off.

- Stand on one or two pillows with both feet and attempt to hold a squat.

- Stand on pillow with one foot.

- Stand on pillow with one foot and try to do a slight squat.

- Do a plank or upright push-up with one arm or hand on each pillow.

- Do the birddog with hand on one pillow and knee on another pillow.

- Do the V-Seat with pillow under buttocks.

- Sit on ground with pillow between knees. Try to hold a V-Seat with the pillow squeezed between knees. This also can be done sitting on a pillow with other pillow between knees.

- Have child lie on back grasping pillow with both hands on the chest. Extend arms out toward the ceiling and toss the pillow. Wait with soft extended arms, catch the pillow and slowly bend arms to bring pillow back to the chest.

- Perform an anterior lunge with lead foot landing on a pillow.

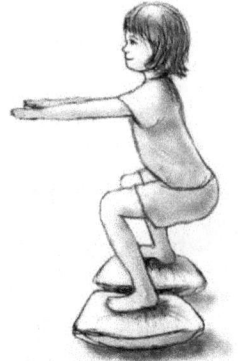

- Lay on back with knees bent, hold the pillow in hands over head, sit up and put the pillow between feet, lay down, now bring the feet over the head and drop the pillow into hands.

- From a kneeling position and upper body in a neutral spine, put a pillow between the feet and squeeze and release.

- Stand with feet shoulder width apart and hold a pillow with both hands in front of face with both elbows pointing outward. Rotate the pillow around the head several times and then reverse the rotation. Keep the head still and do not touch the head with the pillow.

- Grab the pillow with both hands in front of the chest and squeeze and knead the pillow.

- Hold the pillow in front of the body with two hands and try to kick the pillow. Hold the pillow high each time. Look out for furniture!

- Do downward dog or upward dog with a pillow under hands, feet, or hands and feet.

- Perform the mountain pose on a pillow.

- Have child standing tall on one pillow and holding another pillow with both hands high above the head.

- From a crab position with hands or feet on a pillow, walk around a circle moving one hand and foot at a time.

- From a push-up position, with feet or hands on a pillow, walk around a circle moving one hand and foot at a time.

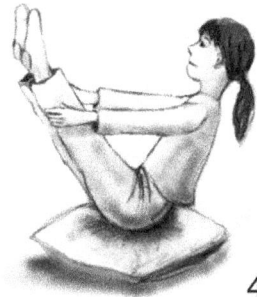

45

SUMO WRESTLER:

Stand up and have the legs wide apart with toes pointed outwards. Put hands on thighs and squat down low.

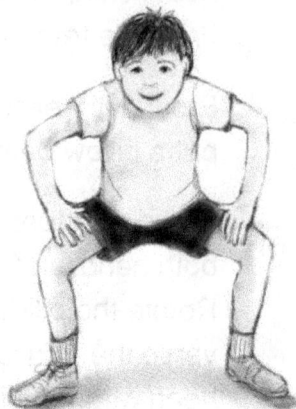

- Take slow steps around the room and add some grunting noises with each step

- Stay in the squat position and perform various arm exercises

- How many steps can be taken before the legs get tired?

- How slow and high can each leg be raised while walking?

- Raise one heel and then the other

- Raise both heels at the same time

- Do punching actions

- Do Sumo jumps-start and end in the sumo position

- How far can the upper body twist without moving feet or knees?

CREATIVE HOPSCOTCH OBSTACLE COURSE:

With chalk, draw one or two side by side blocks in any order on blacktop or cement. Child jumps "hop scotch style" to the end and back.

Optional:

- Keep adding blocks

- When they reach the end they perform an exercise

- Jump with 2 feet in the single block

- Time them

- Try going backwards

- How high can they jump?

- Jump with 2 feet in every box

- Jump only on right or left foot in each block

- To make this more challenging, have the child hold weighted tennis balls

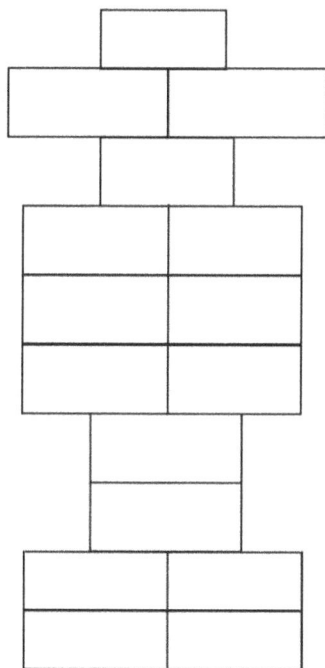

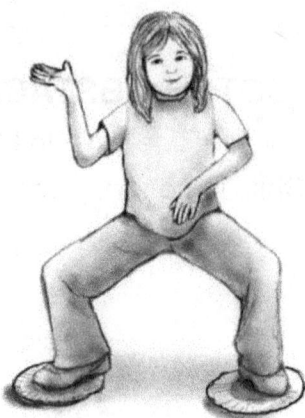

PAPER OR PLASTIC PLATE SHUFFLE: Using paper or plastic plates, this activity should be performed on wall to wall carpet or a grassy area. Be careful of falls or feet out of control.

1. Put each foot on a plate. Walk around carefully by shuffling feet on the paper plates.

2. Try the advanced move of long forward shuffling "cross country skiing" steps and moving the opposite arm forward.

3. Another advanced move is ice skating. Push one foot out to the side at a time.

4. Get in an upright push-up position and put plates under toes. Walk around room using hands only and drag feet.

5. Get in an upright push-up position and put plates under toes. Shuffle feet up toward chest one at a time doing Mountain Climbers.

ANIMALS IN TROUBLE CIRCUIT: Write the animal action on a piece of paper and have child spend about 30 seconds at each station doing activity.

Do the circuit more than once.

- Turtle on it's back slowly moving all four legs
- Frog in a box trying to jump out
- Fish flopping on it's belly on a boat
- Squirrel climbing a very slippery tree
- Bear with his paws stuck in very thick mud
- Baby bird flapping wings and jumping up and down in nest trying to fly
- Dog walking with a sore paw (a 3 paw walk)
- Snake wiggling over a hot road
- Cat scared and curling it's back
- Goat standing on a very small rock
- Wild monkey in cage

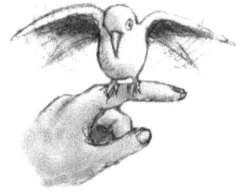

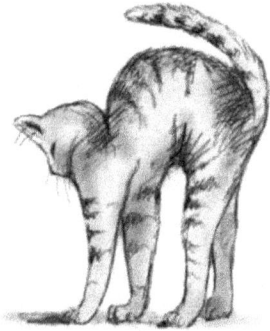

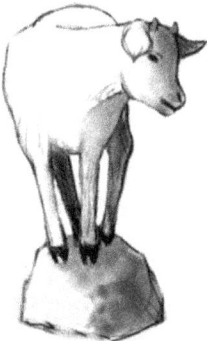

BEAT YOUR BEST: Do several challenges and post them somewhere important. Each time the participant improves their "best", put the new time/number on the challenge board.

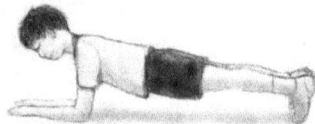

Some suggestions:

- A timed run around the block or to a specific area and back?

- How many times in one minute, can the child lay in a prone position, stand up, jump, and get back down on the ground?

- How long can the plank be held?

- How many times in one minute can the child stand-up/sit-down in a chair?

- How many pushups can be done in 30 seconds?

- How long can the wall squat be held?

- How long can the yoga stick pose be held?

- How fast can the child crawl a short distance?

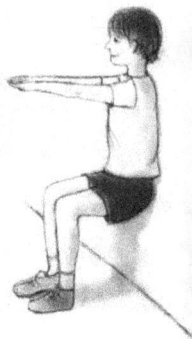

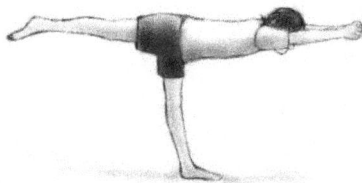

For a better workout:

- Try the best of 3 in one day. Make sure there are rest periods between repeats.
- Try combining several challenges.

MOVEMENT CARDS: Write one fun movement exercise from this book on each index card.

EXAMPLES:

Blastoff, Move like a snake, Sumo wrestler, Volleyball block jump, etc. Child can pick a few cards from the shuffled exercise deck and perform. If you have more participant they can pick cards and then have the option of swapping them without telling each other what they are swapping.

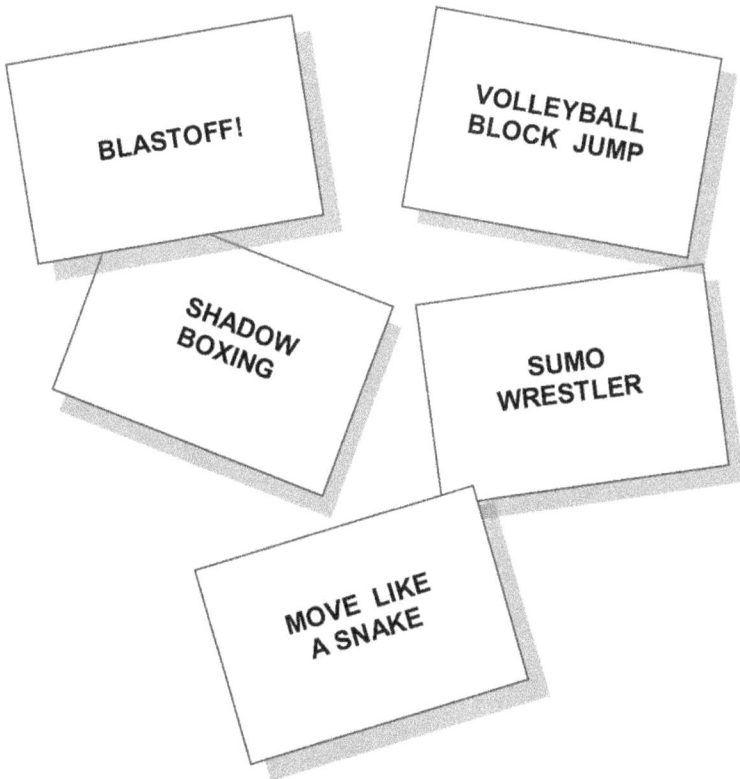

BLASTOFF!

VOLLEYBALL BLOCK JUMP

SHADOW BOXING

SUMO WRESTLER

MOVE LIKE A SNAKE

COMPANY HALT: When marching have the leader chant and the children repeat the chant. Make it fun and make up your own chants: "1, 2, 3, 4, 1, 2, 3, 4, I don't care what people say, I will do this everyday, 1, 2, 3, 4, 1, 2, 3, 4!!" At the end have the children salute.

Options:
- Standing up, march with legs kicking straight and high in front of the body and the opposite arms are also straight and high

- In a downward dog or crab position have the children march in place only using hands

- In a downward dog or crab position have the children march in place only using feet

- In a downward dog or crab position march using hands and feet

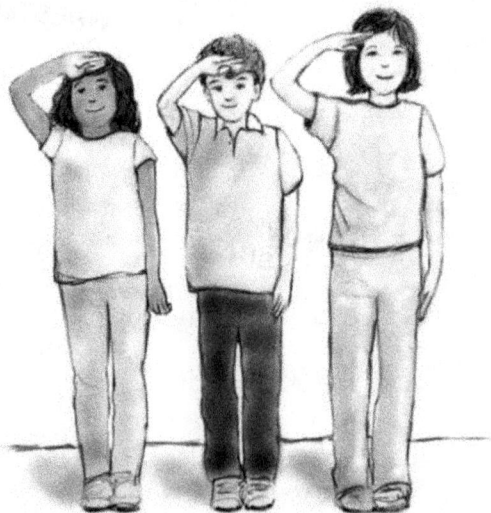

SHADOW BOXING: Go outside on a sunny day and face shadow or stand with a lamp behind you to cast a shadow. Work on various boxing skills at various speeds: Get the hands and arms going, feet moving, ducking punches, bob and weave, etc.

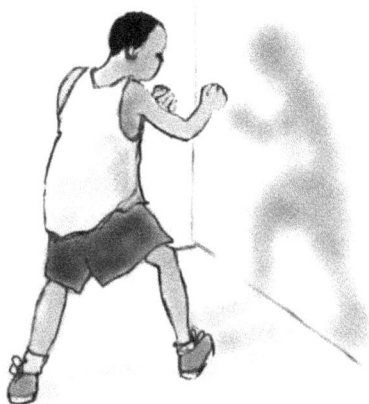

ROLL THOSE TOOTSIES: Place a paper towel under bare foot while sitting. Keep heels on the ground and use only toes and balls of feet. Try to crunch the paper towel into a bundle or move the paper towel forward and back as much as possible. Now do the same with the other foot.

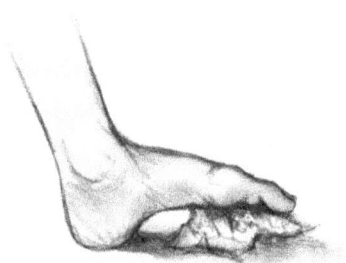

LINE CHALLENGES: Find a line or make one. There are several great challenges to do with a line. Try to do a specific challenge for 15 to 30 seconds. Repeat and try to improve.

Standing sideways with both feet on one side of line

- Jump with both feet over and back.
- Hop on one foot over and back.
- Polka ... leap over the line and have the right foot touch, then the left foot touch, then the right. Now leap to the left and have the left foot touch, then the right, then the left.

Standing sideways with one foot one each side of line

- Jump over line crisscrossing feet. Jump back and uncross.
- Keeping feet on their side of the line, run as fast as possible in place.
- Jump half way around and try to land feet on the opposite side of line.
- Jump all the way around and try to land on the ground in the original take-off spot.
- Jump up and try to click heels and separate feet before landing. Try to do two clicks.

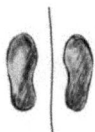

Stand with toes facing line

- Jump over and back with both feet.
- Jump over, slap knees before you landing.
- How many knee slaps can be done before feet hit the ground?

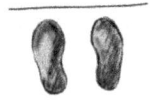

Standing in crab or pushup position with one foot and hand on each side of line

- Go back and forth over the line.
- Touch the line with one hand and then the other.
- Touch the line with one foot and then the other.
- Touch the line with one hand, then one foot, then the other hand and followed by the other foot.
- Touch the line with the opposite foot and hand at the same time.
- Both feet touch the line at the same time.
- Have hands and feet all on the line at the same time and hold balance.

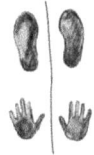

Standing in the crab or pushup position with two feet on one side and two hands on the other side of line

- Go back and forth over the line.
- Touch the line with one hand and then the other.
- Touch the line with one foot and then the other.
- Touch the line with one hand, then one foot, then the other hand and followed by the other foot.
- Both feet touch the line at the same time.

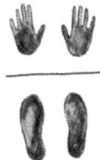

55

EVERYDAY EXERCISE:

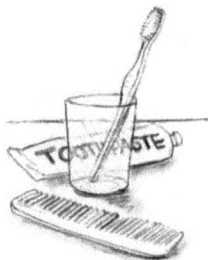

- When brushing teeth put one hand on the sink and raise and drop your heels. Get the heels as high as possible and then slowly bring them back down to floor.

- When in bed do sky walking. Put legs up in the air and pretend feet are slowly walking on the ceiling.

- Sit and stand a few times before sitting down.

- In the car march/walk/jog in place. Do not distract the driver!

- Walk, jog, skip, bike, and find stairs whenever you can.

- Before taking a shower or going in the tub grab a towel with both hands and raise the towel up and down with straight arms. Do this in front and back of the body.

- When on the phone, do squats or lunges.

- Try staying in a plank when reviewing spelling words or reading a few paragraphs.

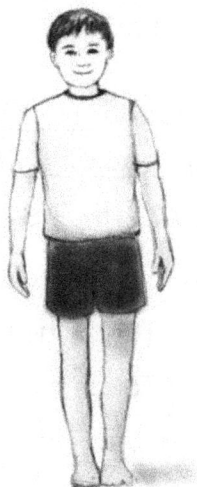

- Do the mountain pose when waiting in line.

- Do homework assignments standing. Place a book on counter/table at chest height. If the table is too low try stacking a few books until desired height.

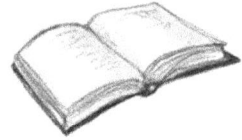

- When sitting raise heels several times and then the toes.

- When looking in a mirror try to become taller with good posture.

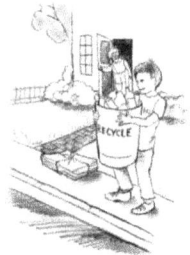

- Exercise and make money - rake leaves, mow lawns, shovel snow, take out trash or become a dog walker, weed a garden.

- March in place when combing hair.

- Do wall push-ups when waiting for the microwave to "beep".

- Walk upstairs two steps at a time.

- Take the stairs instead of elevator. Too high up? Take the stairs until tired and then ride the elevator.

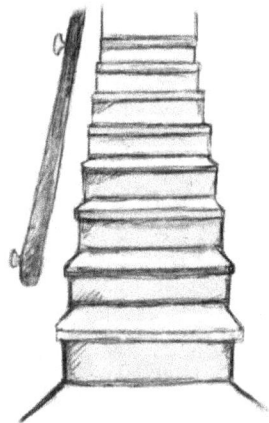

SPORT TRAINING CIRCUIT: Write various sports and exercises on index cards and spread about play area. Have the children do the exercises (no equipment needed) at each station for 30 to 45 seconds. Alternate right and left when the activity is a one sided move.

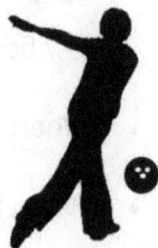

- **Volleyball:** Jump up and block ball

- **Baseball:** Catcher squat and stand to throw ball back to pitcher

- **Yoga:** Prone position, grab feet with hands and try to rock like a boat

- **Lacrosse:** Pickup up ball with stick off of ground - bend your knees and have both of your hands close to ground

- **Karate:** Step and kick foot as high as possible

- **Basketball:** Defense side shuffle back and forth

- **Golf/Ice Hockey/Field Hockey:** Hit the ball or puck

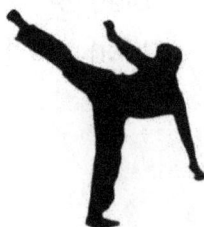

- **Curling:** Sweep the ice as fast as you can

- **Rock climbing:** Reach your hands and your knees up high and climb

- **Surfing:** Lay down on your board and jump up to surfing position

- **Bowling:** Take three steps and roll the ball

- **Table tennis:** Quick steps from side to side and paddle that ball

- **Boxing:** Step and duck that punch

- **Soccer:** Run fast in place

- **Fencing:** Take two steps and lunge

- **Skiing:** Feet together and jump side to side

- **Archer:** Stand sideways and slowly pull back the arrow leading with your elbow

- **Trampoline:** Jumping up in the air see how many different actions you can do with your feet, hands, and whole body ... NO FLIPS

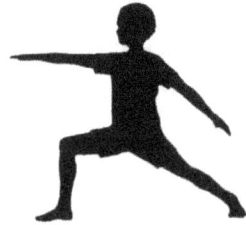

- **Horseback riding:** Feet apart, get into a half squat, and lightly bounce up and down.

- **Discus throw:** Hold onto the discus and spin and throw.

- **Handball:** Slight lunges side to side and hit the ball.

- **Crew:** Sit in V-seat position and use your arms to row the boat.

- **Football:** Run in place as fast as you can, drop quickly to the ground and do 3 pushups, get back up fast and repeat.

- **Luge:** Lay down on back, lift legs, head, and shoulders just a few inches off the ground. Pretend to make turns by slightly moving head and legs sideways.

- **Snowboarder:** Feet shoulder width apart, pointed sideways, knees slightly bent. Jump turn and kick heels up behind.

- **Swimming:** Do a standing butterfly. Make big arm circles and jump up and down.

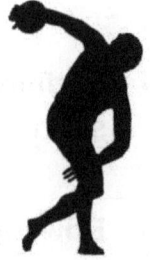

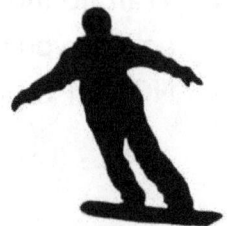

EMERGENCY!: Child marches/jogs in play area and when leader gives signal for **"EMERGENCY"**! they stand still and get ready for action. Leader gives commands with authority! It is easier to teach a few moves at a time.

ACTIONS:

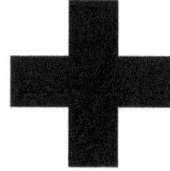

- **"Fire"** stop, drop, and roll

- **"Smoke"** crawl

- **"Man the Lifeboats"** sit and row, move body by stretching legs out in front and then bringing buttocks towards heels.

- **"To the Roof"** pretend to climb a ladder

- **"Which way did they go?"** bird - dog

- **"We need to build a bridge"** have children get in the crab position side by side

- **"Get the Stretcher"** child lays on the ground perfectly still

- **"Flood"** pump the water out by performing push-ups

- **"Man Overboard"** stand on tip toes and pretend the hands are binoculars and cup them around eyes

- **"Earthquake"** quick little jumps

- **"Stop the Traffic"** Warrior II

- **"My Hero"** Warrior I

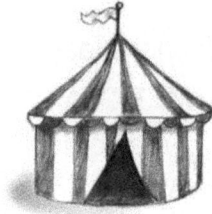

CIRCUS: Place a napkin/tissue on the floor and try to pick it up several different ways.

- Standing on one foot, pick tissue up with hand without putting other foot down

- In an upright push-up position, try to keep the tissue in the air by juggling it back and forth between their hands

- With bare feet, in a squat position pick the tissue up with the toes of one foot and wave it in the air

- In an upright push-up position come down and pick the tissue up with the mouth

- With bare feet pick it up with toes and bring it up to hands, raise the hand higher with each pickup

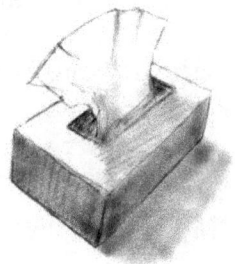

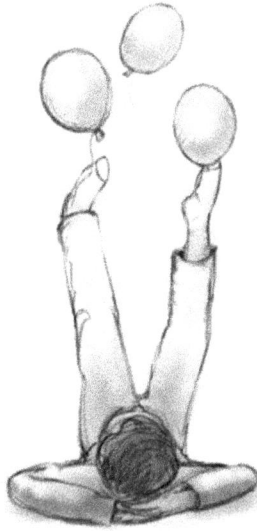

UP, UP & AWAY: Keeping balloons up in the air is a great way to get exercise.

• Try using different body parts (thumbs, elbow, head, knees, sole of foot, etc.)

• Tap back and forth with a partner using the different body parts

• Keep two or three balloons going at the same time

• Keep balloons up while standing, sitting or laying down

• Toss the balloon, go down to a prone position, stand up and toss again

PARTNERS AND MORE

ROCK/PAPER/SCISSORS CHALLENGE: Face partner and both get in a slight squat. Now do one game of Rock/Paper/ Scissors. The loser goes a little deeper in their squat and the winner stays in slight squat. Each time a player loses they go down lower. Play game 5 times and then stand and start over.

To make this more challenging try starting in a slight one-leg squat, wall squat, or lunge.

You can also try a two handed game: right-hand vs partner's left and left-hand vs part-ner's right.

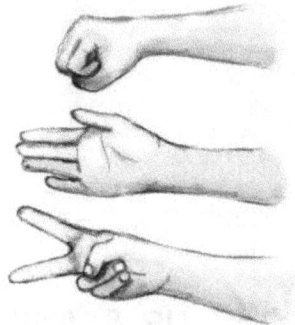

PUSH-UP SOCCER: Two players are in the upward stage of the push-up (modified push-ups can be used) facing each other with 5 or more feet between them. One player has a small foam or yarn ball. Players push the ball back and forth trying to score between opponent's hands. Players may use hands to stop ball. If the ball goes between opponent's hands a goal is scored. If opponent gives up on their push-up position a point is scored by other player. First player to score 5 wins.

Suggestion: Try the push-up soccer game while doing down-ward dog or hands wider apart.

FOOT TAG: Partners stand and face each other holding right hands. Players are not permitted to squeeze, yank, or pull hard on opponent's hand. Both players try to touch the other player's foot with their foot (tap on top) without having their own foot tapped. One point is scored for every tap. After five points are scored, play game holding left hands.

Suggestion: One player is only offense and the other is only defense.

SURVIVOR: Partners do challenges against one another.

- Who can hold the longest one foot squat without moving supporting foot? Try right and then left.

- Who can stay in a v-seat position the longest while sitting on a pillow?

- How many squats can be done with a tissue on the head? Do not touch the paper; if it falls off, stop squatting.

- Who can hold the longest tree pose?

- Who can hold the longest one foot squat while being lightly tickled by partner?

- Who can stay in a v-seat position the longest while tossing and catching a weighted tennis ball.

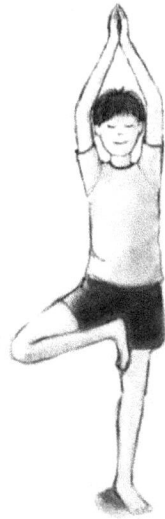

65

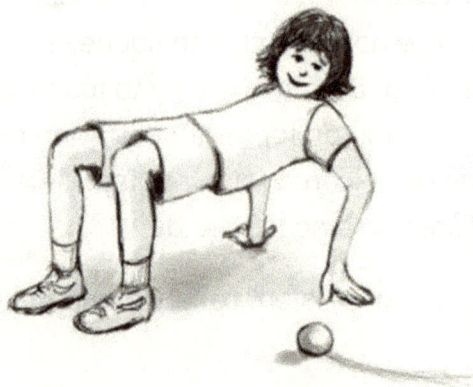

HUMAN BOWLING: One partner has foam ball (bowler) and the other partner (pin) is 25 feet or more away.

The bowler can only roll the ball. The pin must be still in a sideways crab position. Bowler rolls ball aiming at pin's legs/feet and arms/hands. If a limb is hit, the pin must immediately lift that body part off the ground and stay balanced. The pin cannot swat at the ball. If the ball deflects off one limb and hits another, both limbs must be raised. If the ball hits both legs or both arms the game is over and bowler wins. If the pin loses balance the game is over and bowler won. The bowler has only two chances to disable the pin in a game. If the pin can remain balanced after two throws he wins.

This game also can be played with two pins/crabs next to each other.

MEMORY KEEPERS: 2 to 4 partners in a group. From a starting point, Partner A does an aerobic movement to a location and performs an exercise. After the exercise Partner "A" runs back to the starting point and Partner "B" now performs the same path and movements as Partner "A" but adds a new location and exercise. Each time a partner has a turn, they add a new location and exercise. How many locations and exercises can be performed before they forget what to do?

WALL SQUAT CHARADES: Think about all of the things people do while sitting (driving a car, playing video games, doing homework, playing cards, etc). One player performs a wall-squat and acts out a sitting activity. Their partner tries to guess that activity. Take turns until players can no longer think of a sitting activity.

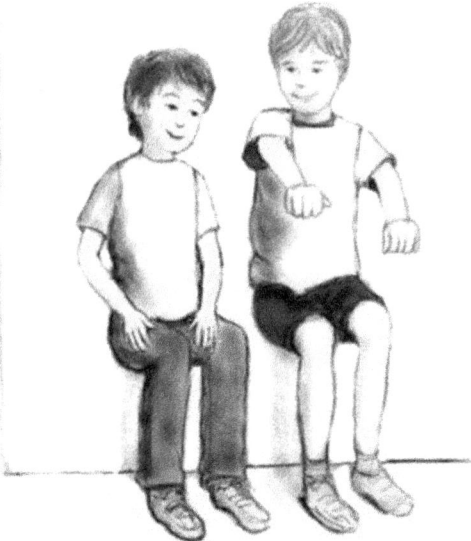

ONE LEG PASS: Face partner at a distance of 10 feet or more and stand on right foot. See how many times the two can pass a ball back and forth without dropping it or touching the left foot on the ground. Switch feet. This is a cooperative activity.

Suggestions:

- Beat highest score
- Throw and catch with one hand
- Do with legs in the Tree Pose
- Standing on left foot, catch, bend down and touch shoe with the ball and then stand up and throw the ball

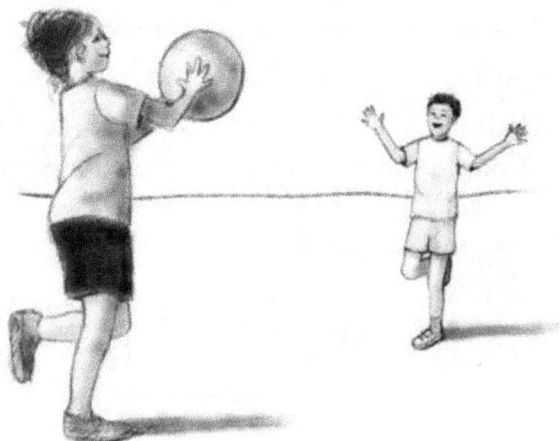

SPORT SIGNALS: The leader will make up a few signals with actions to go with them. Example: "When I touch my nose you do push-ups and when I touch my knees you will run in place as fast as you can." Partner faces leader and looks for signals. Partners take turns being the leader and add a few signals each time.

PARTNER DISTANCE: Partners face each other and are about 5 feet apart. One partner is the leader. Take turns being the leader.

1. The leader walks slowly forward and backwards. When the leader walks forward the follower tries to keep 5 feet away by walking backward. When the leader walks backward the follower now walks forward trying to maintain same distance.

2. Leader does the same but jogs slowly.

3. Leader walks but adds a lunge. When leader lunges the follower must take extra steps back to keep the distance.

4. Do the same drills above, but partners hold the end of a beach towel or 5 foot rope. Try to keep the towel or rope taunt.

• Perform the same as above but partner will slightly move the rope sideways or up and down.

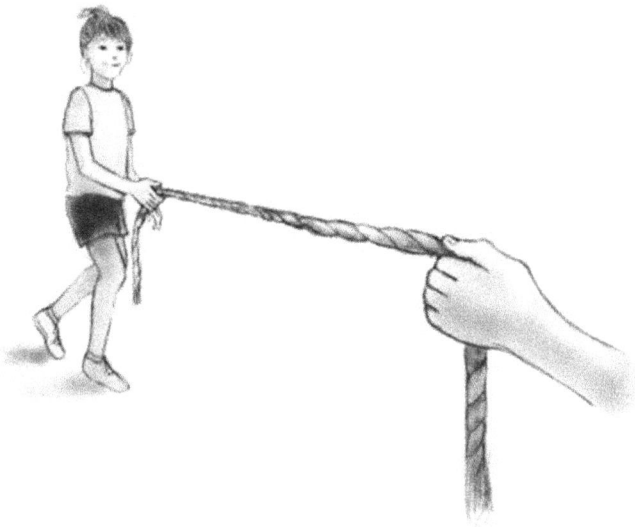

SPIDER WEB: With a partner, make an 8 legged spider. This is done by putting the smaller person in a crab position on the bottom and the larger person in a crab position over the top. The top person is not leaning on the bottom player and their heads and feet are at 90 degrees so that their bodies look like a "+" sign. Now, they must walk around the room pretending to be weaving a web.

Note: It is recommended that the weight difference between the top and bottom child is not significant and same sex also is recommended in a non-family setting.

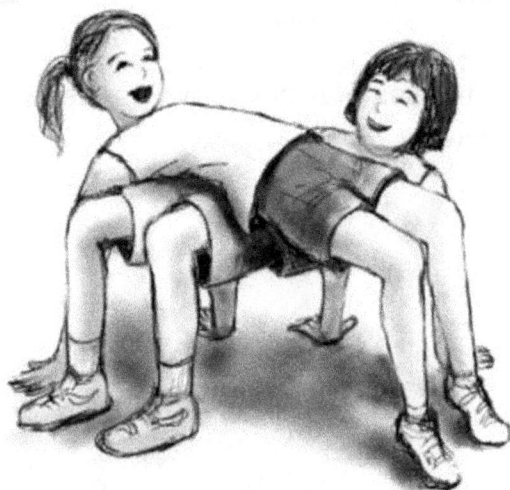

UNDER / AROUND: Partner A is in the downward dog position and does not move. Partner B crawls under partner A and then stands up and runs around partner A and repeats the crawl movement.**

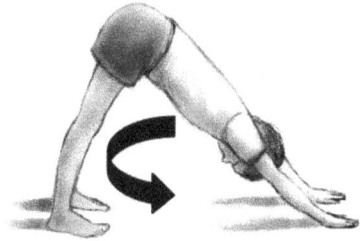

OVER / AROUND: Partner A is in an upward dog position and does not move. Partner B jumps over Partner A's legs and runs around Partner A and repeats movement.**

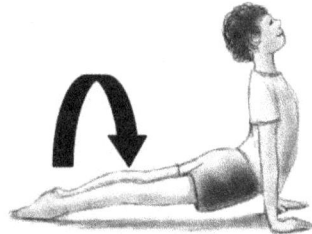

OVER / UNDER: If the children have the skills, alternate the non-moving children on the ground in the downward dog and upward dog position with plenty of space between. Have the runner jump over the legs of the child in the upward dog position and then crawl under the player in the downward position.

**Warning - do not jump over head or spine and do not jump when fatigued.

Have children stay still while in the upward and downward dog position.

DOUBLE BUBBLE TROUBLE: Everyone has a partner. If there is an odd number, this can be done in a group of three. Partners hold hands and pretend they are a bubbles while listening for commands. The leader will give the bubbles a locomotor movement and the bubbles will move around without touching other bubbles or letting go of hands. When a signal is given, the bubbles are to stop and listen. The new command will have them descend or stay in one area various ways (slowly deflate, lightly bounce, twirl around, etc.) Start over with new locomotor movement.

SLAP ME 5: To play this tag game, partners face each other in an upright push-up position to play. Using only hands, players try to touch the top of the other player's hand without their own hand being touched. One point is scored for each tap. If a person gives up their push-up position a point is given to the opponent. First player to score 5 points wins.

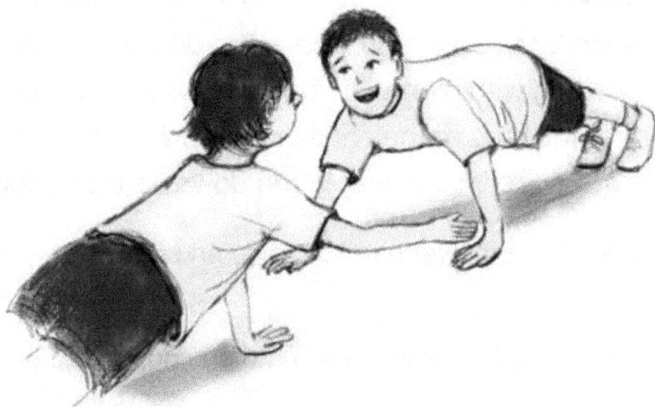

CRUNCH CAPTAIN: Partners are on their backs with knees bent and toes touching each other on the ground. One partner is holding a ball or soft object in their hands. Both partners crunch up, the ball is handed off and then they go back down. Partners continue crunching up and down passing the ball until one can no longer crunch. The remaining "cruncher" is awarded the title Crunch Captain.

Option: Pass object on the outside of knees

V-W: Partners perform V-seat facing each other with toes touching each other in the air to create a "W-seat." While holding the "W-seat" the partners recite the alphabet together until they reach the letters "V-W."

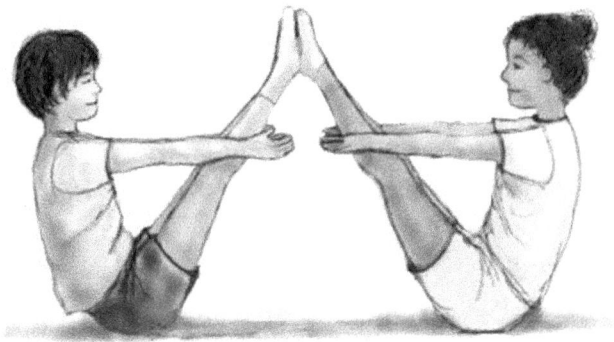

GROUP ACTIVITIES

ARE YOU MY PARTNER?: Write one thing that can be acted out with energy on each index cards. Divide the children into two or more equal groups. Show a different card to each person in one group. Shuffle the cards you used and do the same with the remaining groups. When you say "go" children act out their part and find other people who are acting out the same action. When they find their partners in action they stay together and keep acting.

Some suggestions:

- Man on a pogo stick

- Disco dancing

- Ice hockey player

- Tap dancer

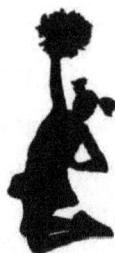

- Cheerleader

- Basketball player

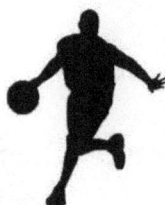

- Drummer marching in a parade

- Ballet dancer

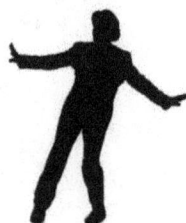

- Robot

TRASH THROW: Gather as many small soft objects as you can (gloves, socks, foam balls, soft hats, yarn balls, etc.) Divide the children into two groups with a middle line that cannot be passed. Have the "trash" (soft objects) on the ground on both sides of the fence (line.) Let the players know that when you say "go" they are going to throw their trash over the fence (line) to the opposite side. They can only pick up, catch and/or throw one item at a time. They must stop immediately when given the signal to stop. The team with the most trash on their side loses.

Option: Perform a lunge when tossing the objects

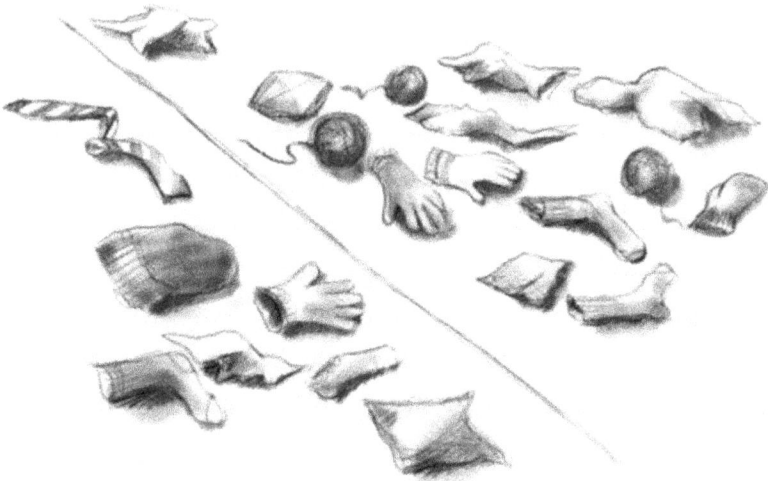

NO BRAKES: Leader is standing on one foot facing other player(s). All players have a paper plate or ball in their hands and are pretending to be driving a car. The object of the game is to follow the leader and not lose your balance. Both the leader and the partner's supportive foot cannot move and foot off the ground cannot touch the ground. Leader will make various turns (fast, slow, sharp, long) with arms and upper torso and partner or group is to follow.

To make this more difficult, players can:
- Hold onto a weighted tennis ball
- Stand on balls of feet and toes
- Have the legs in the tree pose position

EXERCISE TAG: Tag games are a great way to get children moving. Tag games can increase aerobic endurance and more. Instead of children freezing when tagged, have them perform an exercise or silly move. To prevent the children from becoming tripping hazards, keep the children in an upright position while they are performing their exercise or silly movement. Make one person "it" for every 7 or 8 people you have in the group.

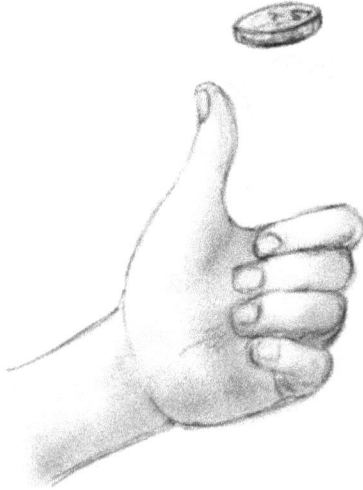

HEADS/TAILS: Standing in the middle of a play area with one end of area designated as "heads" and the other as "tails." The leader will flip a coin after the children guessed the outcome by running to the selected area. Those who guessed wrong are eliminated and move to the side by the leader and perform an exercise. Those who guessed right return to the center and continue the game. Keep repeating game until there is one remaining player.

GRAB THE TAIL: Everyone has a tail (handkerchief, sock, or piece of material) tucked lightly into the back of their pants. On the signal to start, everyone tries to steal someone's tail without their own tail being snatched. Only one tail can be taken at a time and players cannot hold onto their own tail. When a tail is taken, the player without a tail still can play. The player who stole the tail now has two tails side by side on his/her backside. Game ends when leaders wants it to end and the player with the most tails wins.

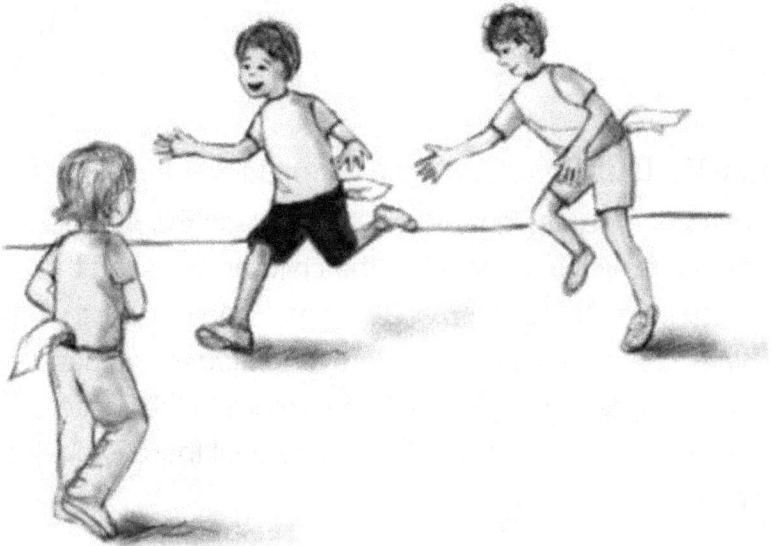

CRAZY BALL: Scatter all types of balls and soft objects around playing area. On a signal everyone runs to an object, throws it up into the air and catches it three times and then proceeds to another object or ball. Do this for 2 minutes or more and have them count how many different objects they threw.

Options:

- Clap hands 1x, 2x, and then 3x before each catch

- Touch knees before catch

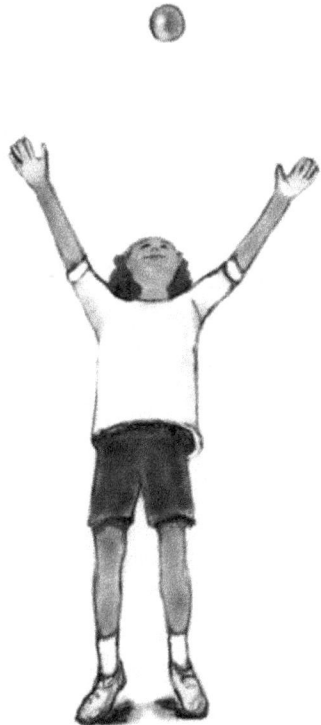

- Throw ball up and touch ground before it is caught

- Throw ball up and do a jumping jack

- Throw ball up lay down and stand up

- Throw ball up and turn half way around before catch

- Throw and turn all the way around before the catch

THE WAVE: Everyone knows the wave from sporting events. Now, try this several ways with your group.

Suggestions:

- Push-up Wave

- Squat Wave

- Lunge Wave

- Prone Position to Standing Wave

- Supine Position to Standing

- Downward Dog to Upward Dog

Remember, do the wave going up and then back down. This also can be done running, skipping, dribbling, etc across a field to a line.

Options:

- Once the wave has been accomplished, have the last person run to the opposite end and be the first person

- Time the children and see if they can go faster

- Try to make it perfect

- Do it in a circle and keep it going round and round

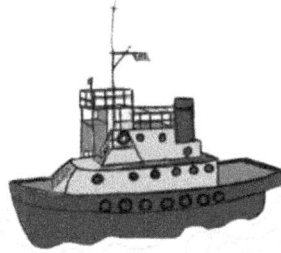

LET'S PRETEND: Many times when young children are running in movement games they have a habit of not watching where they are going. Try working on spatial awareness with the following:

Child will move when told and will stop immediately when signal is given. They can go anywhere in a designated area. You can start with slower motions and if they are successful, have the movement progress to a faster movement (for example: a horse walking, trotting, galloping, running and jumping over fences). Warn children if they do not watch where they are going, they might have to go back to the dock, barn, garage, etc. All movements are done in an upright position.

START AS:	PROGRESS TO:
Slow moving tug boat................ ..	Coast Guard rescue boat
Horse walking in a parade	Horse running and jumping fences
Person driving car in school zone....	Police car chasing criminal
Skating on a pond	Olympic speed skater
Eagle soaring in the sky...............	Hummingbird, fast flapping wings & dodging moves

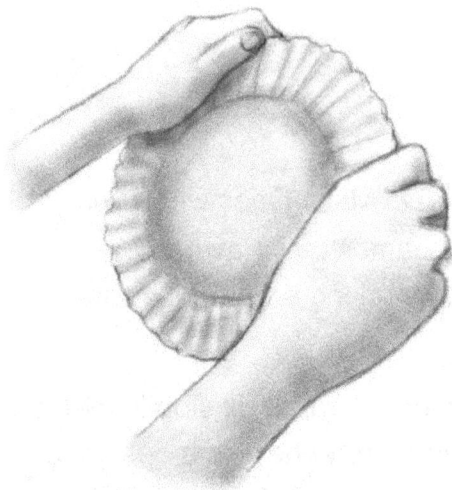

MECHANIC: Spread out several obstacles on the ground or use lines. Break everyone into groups of 4 to 6. One person in the group is the mechanic and the others are cars. If available, have the cars hold paper plates or balls and pretend they are holding steering wheels. The cars are unable to turn and can only jog, skip or march in one direction. When a car comes to an obstacle (cones, chairs, lines, walls, other car, etc.), they cannot turn and must jump up and down in their spot shouting for their mechanic by name "Mechanic Jasmine, Mechanic Jasmine." The mechanic runs to their car in need and turns the steering wheel . The car now continues in the direction they were turned until they run into another obstacle.

CRAB TAG: Players are in crab position about 5 feet apart. On the signal "go," players are trying to touch opponent's lower leg (knee to foot) without their own leg's being tagged. One point is scored for each successful touch. The buttocks cannot dip down and touch the ground. This game can be played with more than 2 players. Warn players to be careful not to step on hands of players.

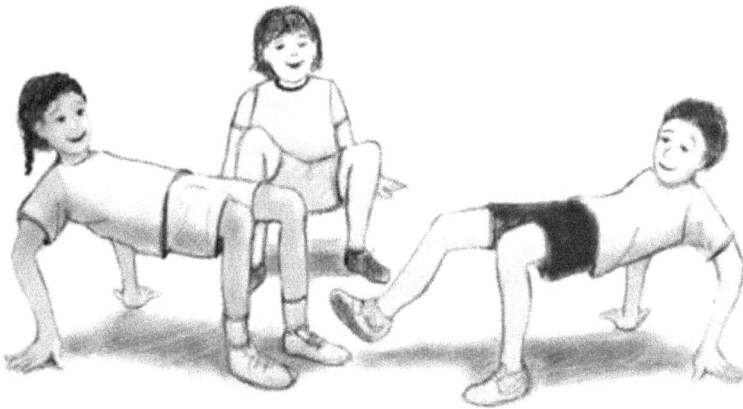

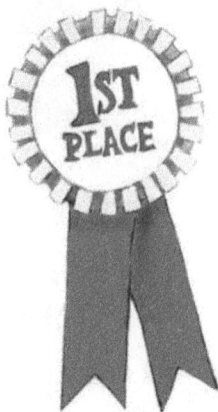

ON YOUR OWN

Take the ideas from this book and expand!

- **CIRCUIT TRAINING:** Mix-up a child's favorite activity with ones that are essential for their fitness needs.

- **TAG:** Tag games are a great way to get children moving. Tag games can increase aerobic endurance, improve agility and more. There are so many variations of this old favorite. I prefer games that keep everyone moving or get them quickly back into the game.

- **CHANGE:** Change where, when and how you exercise. Try some of the exercises in a pool. Go to a local high school stadium/lighthouse/monument and climb the stairs. Pretend to climb and descend the Statue of Liberty (354 steps to crown) using your own staircase. Go for a bike ride or take a local hiking trail. Go to a local fitness class, dance class, or try a new sport. Take a night walk with the family when there is a full moon.

- **CROSS TRAINING:** Do not do the same type of exercise all the time. Variety is good for the mind and body.

- **OBSTACLE COURSE:** Children love to crawl under, jump over, go through, and climb obstacles.

- **SPORT SPECIFIC:** If you want to introduce your child to a specific sport movement or you are a coach, modify some of the games in this book for drills. Remove movements and substitute shooting, dribbling, cradling, swimming, footwork, or other sport specific skills.

- **MOTIVATION:** Keep a log, set goals, chart progress, and/or find inspirational quotes.

- **PRESIDENT CHALLENGE AWARDS:** Receive fitness awards by logging onto www.presidentschallenge.org . Child will have their personal activity log for every activity from bike riding to squats. When they reach a designated level they can apply for various awards.

- **RELAY RACES:** Mix the talent up and add various movements to make it fun and challenging.

- **FRIENDLY COMPETITIONS:** Have a family Olympics or street champions, or fitness party.

- **INVOLVE THE CHILD:** Responsibility in one's own fitness is a way of life. Have the children move the cones, set up the boundaries, carry the balls, clear the area, enter their activities in logs, and make the fitness cards.

CREATING AN EXERCISE PLAN

Planning and using an exercise chart can be helpful. Decide ahead of time what activities will be used for the warm-up and cool-down, and what game(s) will be played.

Ask yourself ahead of time:

- Are there space challenges for these activities?

- Is there a need for cones or markers for off limit areas?

- How much time will be needed for instruction and activity?

- Is the activity age appropriate?

- Do the children have the fitness level to perform the activities?

- What equipment is needed for the activities?

- Should a focus on a fitness component (strength, endurance, speed, balance, etc) be considered?

- What safety precautions should be taken?

- Is the activity challenging?

EXERCISE PLAN / WORKOUT CHART

Warm - up:

Equipment:

Time:

Games / Activities:

Equipment:

Time:

Cool - down:

Equipment:

Time:

Goals:

Tear-Out & make copies to keep track of your child's fitness progress.

HEALTHY DIET & FITNESS

A healthy diet is part of fitness. What children eat is an important factor in their health.

The following websites contain activities for children to learn about nutrition and fitness.

- The US Department of Agriculture: www.mypyramid.gov
- The Canadian Government: www.cflri.ca
- The American Council for Fitness and Nutrition: www.acfn.org

For more information about nutrition and diet go to the American Dietetic Association's website www.eatright.org .

A child's body needs the proper type of fuel, that means the right amount of calories and nutrients from healthy food. Hydration from water also is essential. When possible, try to avoid empty calorie food such as soda pop and non-nutritional snacks.

Introducing new foods to a child should be done slowly. Some of the more common foods that cause allergies are: cow's milk, peanuts, tree nuts, wheat, soy, eggs, shellfish, and fish.

HEALTHY FOOD HINTS

- Try yogurt instead of syrup on whole wheat pancakes or waffles.

- Soda pop can have the equivalent of 14 teaspoons of sugar in 16 oz.

- Go to favorite fast food restaurant's website to see calories, fat, fiber, etc. of items.

- Look at food labels before picking items.

- Wash and freeze grapes for a quick refreshing snack.

- Put yogurt or real juice in ice cube trays for a frozen treat.

- If a child loves unhealthy cereal, try mixing it with a healthy cereal.

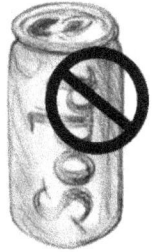

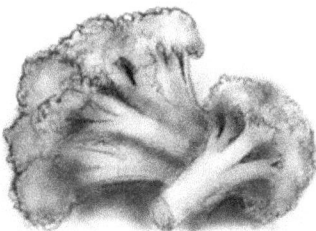

- Try unsweetened applesauce in place of butter.

- Have children make their own trail mix: various cereals, soy nuts, raisins and other dried fruit, dark chocolate, and nuts.

- Bake, steam, grill, broil, boil, or eat raw instead of frying.

- Avoid ingredients that end in the letters "-ose". Various sugars end in these letters.

- Spray salad dressing instead of pouring.

- Mix boiled potatoes with boiled cauliflower to make healthy mashed potatoes. Substitute greek yogurt or low fat plain yogurt for milk, butter, and/or sour cream.

- Use yogurt as a dip for veggies or fruit.

- Add a few nuts to top of salad, baked potatoes, cereal, yogurt, steamed vegetables and more.

- Mix real juice with club soda.

- When ordering pizza, skip the meat toppings and order vegetable toppings.

- Keep vegetables clean/cut and ready at eye level in the refrigerator.

- Avoid food that has sugar, fructose or, corn syrup among first 4 ingredients on food label.

- Try to purchase whole grain products instead of those containing white flour.

- Peel and freeze bananas. Make a milkshake with frozen bananas, vanilla extract, and skim milk.

- Try the following recipe instead of french fries; Preheat oven to 375 degrees, cut potatoes in wedges or slices, toss lightly with olive oil, bake in roasting pan until the bottom of potatoes are brown, turn and cook for additional 5 to 15 minutes. Also try this with sweet potatoes or other vegetables

- A standard favorite for children to make is **"Ants on a Log"** : Celery filled with peanut butter and topped with raisins. Add red ants - dried cranberries or dried cherries. Add dirt and rocks – crushed nuts or seeds. Put peanut butter and raisins on broccoli and have **"Ants in a Tree"**. Try using a piece of lettuce and have **"Ants on a Leaf"**.

- Fun food challenge: Place several healthy bite size items on a plate and child picks up the food using one chopstick in each hand.

- Do not read the front of packages! Just because they say "natural" or "healthy" does not mean that it is good for you. Read the ingredients on the back!

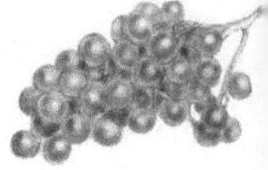

- Grow a garden with your child. This might be a big backyard garden or a little window herb garden. Children usually are enthusiastic about eating food that they helped grow. Sprinkle the herbs on chicken, vegetables, or fish and watch the pride and joy as they eat their food.

- Have children help prepare healthy meals or pack lunch.

- Put a healthy meal in a backpack and walk to a local park or scenic locations.

- Put slices of real fruit in a nice cold glass of water.

- Buy real cheese products instead of the wording "processed product, imitation, food, or spread."

- Purchase peanut butter that does not contain sugar or salt. Example: Crazy Richard's Peanut Butter.

- Tortilla Pizza: Whole wheat tortilla topped with a little tomato sauce, thin sliced vegetables and a little cheese. Bake for a few minutes on a cookie sheet.

- Replace sugary jams and jellies with real fruit in a peanut butter and jelly sandwich. Try sliced bananas, strawberries, or kiwi.

- When purchasing lunchmeat, buy one that does not contain fillers, MSG, extenders or artificial colors. Example: Dietz & Watson premium meats.

- Instead of chips, try sliced apples, or pears. Serve with salsa, yogurt, real cheese, guacamole, peanut butter, or almond butter.

- Cook skinned chicken in crock-pot with salsa and serve over rice or grains.

- Cut vegetables in small pieces and slow cook or puree to thicken soups. Try sweet potatoes, carrots, or cauliflower.

- Puree leftover cooked vegetables and add to spaghetti sauce.

- Add uncooked oatmeal or multi-grain hot cereal to pancakes, muffins, cookies, streusel topping as a substitute for some of the flour. The oatmeal or cereal can also be used to thicken soup.

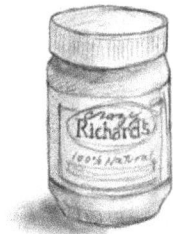

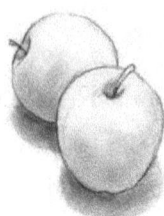

- Involve children in the cooking process: making grocery list, reading recipes, washing fruit & vegetables, shredding lettuce & greens, measuring, stirring, timing, and serving. Share the pride they will have watching everyone enjoy their meal.

- If the child is a picky eater, tell them to eat a "no thank you helping" of the healthy food. This is just a spoonful or more.

- Pick dark chocolate over milk, or white chocolate.

- For a sweet snack, try dark chocolate covered nuts or dried fruit.

- Healthier pancake recipe: Mix 1 cup oatmeal or multi-grain hot cereal, 1 cup whole wheat flour, 1 tablespoon baking soda, 1 tablespoon sugar with 1 beaten egg, 1 mashed banana, and 1 cup of milk or enough to make the thickness you desire. Pour onto a lightly oiled frying pan and serve with yogurt or topping of choice.

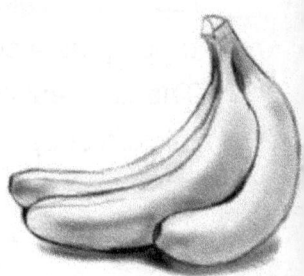

- Healthier chicken tenders: Preheat oven to 350 degrees. Smear plain low fat yogurt all over skinless chicken pieces, pour ¼ cup whole wheat flour and ¾ cup whole wheat breadcrumbs in bowl or zip-lock bag, add desired seasoning (salt, pepper, Italian, poultry, thyme, etc.) and coat chicken with mixture. Spray or lightly coat oil on cookie sheet, place chicken on sheet and bake until done. You also can use this recipe for fish or pork.

- Make a smoothie with vanilla yogurt, berries, banana and a few ice cubes in a blender.

- Make a parfait for breakfast or snack. Layer yogurt and berries in a tall glass and top the parfait with nuts and/or cereal.

- For a healthy dessert, barbecue fruit on the grill. Try pineapple, apples, pears, peaches and more. Put a spoonful of yogurt on top and sprinkle with cinnamon.

- Food art project: Let the children be creative making an edible art project using healthy food . Start with applesauce, hummus, mashed cauliflower, mashed sweet potatoes, yogurt or peanut butter. Top with peas, corn, sliced vegetables, seeds, nuts, cheese and/or fruit.

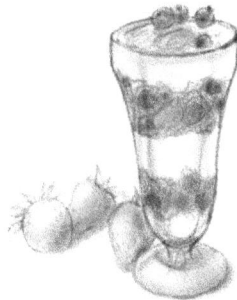

WEIGHT CONTROL

If a child has been diagnosed as overweight, the suggestions listed below may help. When it comes to exercise, body weight and energy balance are directly connected. In order to lose weight the child needs to eat less, eat healthier and exercise. Muscles burn more calories that fat.

PORTION SIZE

Portion size can be a problem with many families. A fun way to memorize serving size is below.

One Serving size:

- Vegetable and chopped fruit = size of adult fist
- Cooked pasta = one ice cream scooper full
- Cheese = pair of dice
- Meat, fish or poultry = deck of cards
- Peanut butter = ping-pong ball
- Butter = dime
- Dry cereal = tennis ball
- Cooked cereal = ½ tennis ball
- Cooked beans = baseball
- Pretzels = ½ tennis ball

WEIGHT CONTROL HINTS

- The bathroom scale is not always a true measurement of fat loss. Monitor progress by taking body measurements and/or how clothes fit.

- Try to eat 3 times slower.

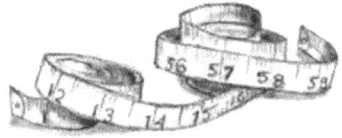

- Take small bites and count chews.

- There are 3,500 calories in a pound. Try eating 500 less calories a day to lose a pound a week. Add exercise and more weight will be lost.

- Put the fork down between small bites.

- Buy child's size portion when indulging in something fattening.

- Eat a healthy breakfast. Food in the morning can increase the metabolism.

- Try horseradish, yogurt, sugar-free applesauce, hummus, mustard, lemon, salsa, relish in place of butter or mayonnaise.

- Take the skin off the chicken and turkey.

- Use smaller plates for meals.

- Do not eat dinner family style, put food on the plate and the extra food away from the table. Vegetables can be served family style.

- Try lemon, vinegars, no fat yogurt or salsa instead of salad dressings.

- Replace that bagel and cream cheese with a whole wheat english muffin and cottage cheese.

- Have open-face sandwiches instead of top and bottom.

- Drink skim milk instead of whole or 2% milk.

- Eat bran flakes instead of bran muffins.

- Try using chopsticks instead of fork.

- Cook oatmeal, cinnamon & sugar free applesauce in micro-wave in place of cinnamon bun.

- Exercise instead of eating when watching TV.

- Try using the opposite hand when using a fork or spoon ... do not do this with hot or sloppy food!

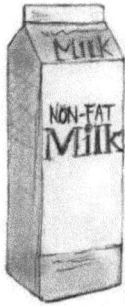

- Keep a food log.

- Substituting water for soda, juice or drinks can save thousands of calories in a year.

- Switch from cream based soups to vegetable-based soups

- Switch from premium ice cream to light ice cream.

- Craving a treat? Cut the normal portion in half and take very small bites.

- Limit TV time.

- Make an egg salad or tuna fish salad with drained low-fat yogurt or greek yogurt, and relish to taste.

- Do not eat while watching TV.

- Offer limited portion snacks a few times a day. Try vegetables, nuts, part-skim string cheese, air popped popcorn, fruit, or hard boiled eggs.

- Use salsa as a dip for celery or carrots.

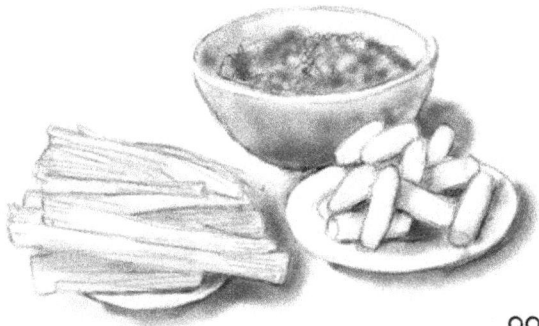

SLEEP AND WELL - BEING

Sleeping is an essential part of fitness and well-being. The right amount of sleep is needed for growth and development and helps a child stay alert. Exercise will energize many children and it is not recommended that they exercise right before bed time. The National Sleep Foundation states that children from age 5 to 12 should receive 10 to 11 hours of sleep every night.

Sleep Tight Hints:

- Have a routine before bedtime; this might be a bath, book, soft music, laying out clothes for the next day or just time to have a nice conversation

- Make the bedroom noise free

- Make the bedroom as dark as possible

- Visualizing a calm and peaceful environment helps many children sleep peacefully

- Select bed-clothes for comfort not style

- Relaxation through slow deep breathing is a great way to start the night in bed

- Keep rigorous exercise earlier in the day

- Maintaining a consistent sleep schedule is helpful for most children

FITNESS LOG

Date:

Exercises:

Aerobic:

Muscular:

Flexibility:

Other - free play, sport, recreational:

Nutrition:

Breakfast:

Lunch:

Dinner:

Snacks:

Sleep:

Hours:

Tear-Out & make copies to keep track of your child's fitness progress.

FITNESS RESOURCES

- The Centers for Disease Control and Prevention: BMI (Body Mass Index) Percentile Calculator for Children: www.cdc.gov

- The President's Challenge: A Physical Fitness Test that is often given in schools: www.presidentschallenge.org

- National Sleep Foundation: Information about sleep and sleep disorders. www.sleepfoundation.org

- American Red Cross: First Aid, CPR & AED certification programs designed to give you skills that can save a life. www.redcross.org

- National Center for Sport Safety: Courses offered for coaches, youth volunteer, and teachers to help avoid preventable injuries. www.sportsafety.org

- US Department of Agriculture: Information about dietary needs for children: www.mypyramid.gov

- The American Council for Fitness and Nutrition: www.acfn.org

- American Dietetic Association: www.eatright.org

- The Canadian Government: www.cflri.ca

GLOSSARY

- **Abduction** - movement of a body part away from body's midline.
- **Acceleration** - increase of speed or velocity
- **Adduction** - movement of a body part toward body's midline.
- **Aerobic Exercise** - activities that increase the demand of oxygen **over an extended time.**
- **Agility** - ability to change direction swiftly while maintaining control and balance of one's body.
- **Anterior** - forward or to the front
- **Atrophy** - reduction of muscle size due to inactivity.
- **Auditory Learning** - understand from hearing.
- **Balance** - within the bodies base of support while maintaining center of gravity.
- **Ballistic Exercise** - bouncing.
- **Calcium** - a nutrient found in foods that help to build and maintain bones.
- **Calisthenics** - exercise workout for specific muscular conditioning using resistance.
- **Calorie** - A unit of energy stored in food and available to the body for functions. One pound equals 3,500 calories.
- **Cardiovascular** - pertaining to blood, heart, lungs, and blood vessels.
- **Cool Down** - slowing down gradually after intense exercising.
- **Co-ordination** - ability to perform complex tasks, improved neuro-muscular efficiency.
- **Circuit Training** - moving quickly from one exercise to another.

GLOSSARY

- **Cross Training** - variation of workouts
- **Decelerate** - to slow down
- **Defense** - protect , thwart attack
- **Duration** - exercise session length.
- **Elevation** - to raise muscles, bones or body part.
- **Empty Calories** - food that is void of nutrients, proteins, minerals, and vitamins
- **Extension** - motion that increases the angle between two bones
- **Fatigue** - diminished capacity for work as a result of exertion
- **FITT Principle** - Frequency, Intensity, Time, and Type of exercise
- **Flexibility** - range of motion of a joint
- **Flexion** - bending the joint between two bones and decreasing the angle between the two bones
- **Frequency** - how often the exercise is performed
- **Heat Exhaustion** - usually result from intense exercise in a hot, humid environment. Characterized by profuse sweating, drop in blood pressure, light-headedness, nausea, vomiting, decreased coordination, and often fainting.
- **Heat Cramps** - forceful and painful muscle contractions caused by heat, dehydration and/or poor conditioning
- **Heat Stroke** - a medical emergency caused by a very hot environment. Symptoms include warm flushed skin, the victim is not currently sweating and usually has a very high body temperature.
- **Hop** - start with one foot and end on same foot
- **Intensity** - level of strength, energy, or difficulty performed in an exercise

GLOSSARY

- **Isometric Exercise** - movement against an immovable force. Muscle length remains the same
- **Isotonic Exercise**- strength training exercises and/or equipment that provide a constant resistance throughout the range of movement
- **Joints** - meeting place of two or more bones
- **Jump** - start on two feet and end on two feet or one foot
- **Kinesthetic Learning** - understand from doing
- **KIS** - Keep it simple
- **Lateral** - to the side
- **Leap** - start with 1 foot and end on the other foot
- **Locomotor Movement** - moving from one area to another. Example: jogging, marching, skipping, walking, hopping, etc.
- **Mobility** - the extent of joint movement before being restricted by surrounding tissue
- **Muscular Endurance** - the ability of the muscle to perform repetitive work over a prolonged period of time
- **Muscular Strength** - the maximum force that can be exerted by a muscle or muscle group
- **Neutral Spine** - a spine with correct upright posture
- **Nutrients** - substance found in foods that provide energy to help growth and maintain and repair body tissues
- **Offense** - to attack, attempt to score
- **Plyometrics** - exercises that maximize the stretch reflex to teach muscles to produce maximum force faster. Usually utilizing sport specific hops, bounds, and depth jumps.

GLOSSARY

- **Posterior** - behind or to the back
- **Power** - exerting great force quickly
- **Prone** - lying facing downward
- **Protein** - A calorie containing food nutrient that provides the building blocks for the body
- **ROM** - (Range of motion) . The number of degrees that a joint will allow one of its segments to move.
- **Rate of Perceived Exertion (RPE)** - How difficult one believes they are exercising
- **Repetitions (REPs)** - How often you repeat an exercise continuously
- **Resting Heart Rate (RHR)** - The number of heart beats per minute when the body is completely at rest
- **RICE** - treatment to perform immediately after an injury: Rest, Ice, Compression and Elevation
- **Set** - a group of repetitions of an exercise
- **Soft Joints** - relaxed, slightly bent
- **SOM** - (Speed of motion). How fast an exercise is performed.
- **Speed** - ability to move the body across space quickly
- **Static Stretch** - a relaxed low-force and long duration stretch
- **Stability** - ease of which balance is maintained
- **Supine** - lying face upward
- **Visual Learning** - understanding from seeing

NOTES

NOTES

NOTES

INDEX

ABOUT THE AUTHOR AND ARTIST

Jane and I were born in the same small hospital just days apart. We both were high school athletes growing up just miles away from each other; we attended the same college; but, we did not know each other until we started fencing in our early forties. We shared the same enthusiasm and joy of competition. Even when fencing against one another, the joy of competing was more important than the outcome.

However, Jane was more skilled than I. On Jane's 50th birthday she won her first of more than 15 National Fencing Championships. I went surfing on mine!

Not only is Jane an accomplished artist and illustrator, in 2005 she won the World Championship for Veteran's Women's Sabre. She still is competing and is rated as one of the top Veteran Women's Sabre fencers in the world.

Ever since I was a young girl I have been active. Competing in high school, club, college and/or nationally in field hockey, lacrosse and fencing. I have surfed, skied, played water polo, dabbled in most sports and have even tried street luging while attending a workshop at the Lake Placid Olympic Training Center.

I always have attended seminars, conferences, and workshops pertaining to sports, physical fitness, sports medicine, personal training, and/or sport safety gaining knowledge and discovering different techniques to get and stay fit. I was a Physical Education teacher for 30 years and have seen the physical conditioning of our children steadily decline. I realized something should be done but knew if it was not fun, it would not work.

With these experiences, my years of education, and being a Personal Trainer I have written this book with hope it will help to keep both you and your children fit as well as build a stronger bond that comes with being active together.

Sue Tracey

Acknowledgements

We want to acknowledge the following people
who supported us in many ways in the creation of this book.

Mike Tracey, Elaine Rode, and Deb Stopak.

Both of us would also like to mention our sons,
Doug Tracey and Josh Tartaglione,
who have inspired us to become the best we can be.

Sue and Jane

~~FINISH LINE~~

There is no finish line in fitness training. Staying healthy and fit is a lifetime commitment.

The habit of exercising and eating healthy for life, is one of the greatest gifts you can give a child.